PMH-BC Study Guide

By Newstone Test Prep

Table of Contents

****The exam simulator instructions, additional tests and other files can be downloaded by using the QR code located on the last page of this book.**

If the QR code does not work for you, please contact us at info@newstonetestprep.com and mention the title of this book.

Background

Before taking the national certification exam, you should review the General Testing and Renewal Handbook found at nursingworld.org. This handbook contains information on the test content, sample questions, testing sites, what to expect on the day of the exam, etc.

The total time for the exam is four hours. This time includes check-in, instructions, and a practice session on the computer. After you finish the test, you will complete a brief survey that will provide feedback to the American Nurses Credentialing Center (ANCC) for quality improvement.

How To Prepare for the Exam

Control Your Anxiety

If you feel anxiety before the certification exam, this is completely normal. To reduce your anxiety, you can remind yourself that the program you participated in was designed to prepare you for this exam. The study plan you develop before the exam and the care with which you review the material will help you feel more confident in your abilities.

Set Reasonable Expectations

Don't set too high expectations of yourself. You don't have to pass the exam with a perfect score. This exam is made to evaluate readiness for entry-level practice. It will not assess you on atypical cases and rare diseases. As you prepare, focus on the most common diagnoses and therapy.

Prepare Yourself Mentally and Physically

It is important to take good care of yourself as you prepare to take the exam. Remember to eat nutritious food and get appropriate amounts of sleep and exercise.

Access Current Knowledge

Carefully review the table of contents in this book, as well as the test content found at nursingworld.org. Ask yourself if you know these topics well enough. You can take a review course to assess your mastery of the content. Schedule your review course so you have enough time to work on any weaknesses you might discover. Remember, the review course should help you identify points of weakness as well as areas of strength.

Strategies Before the Exam

Incorporate practice tests into your study plan to help you get accustomed to the test format and alleviate anxiety. Practice tests can also improve your exam-taking skills.

Get familiar with your test-taking style. Some people tend to rush through the exam and don't thoroughly read the questions, while others tend to get stuck on questions. You should spend approximately 45 to 60 seconds per question. Make sure to read all answer choices carefully.

As you take the practice tests and the exam itself, try not to overanalyze things. The person who wrote the test assumes that all the information given is enough to answer the questions. Therefore, information that is not included is not relevant to the answer. Read all the answers carefully. Only one answer is correct. If two answers seem correct, you must determine the best answer for the specific questions.

Chapter 1: Developmental Stages

Erik Erikson's Stages of Psychosocial Development

Erik Erikson's stages of psychosocial development were created in the 1950s. They consist of eight stages of ego development characterized by psychosocial crises (basic conflicts) that reflect the needs of the individual and conflict with the needs of society. The resolution of a crisis can cause either personal growth or psychosocial regression. An individual who completes each stage acquires basic virtues that can be used to resolve the next crises. An individual who fails to resolve a crisis may develop a maladaptive personality and unhealthy sense of self.

Stage One: Trust versus Mistrust (Birth to about 18 Months)

This is the first stage in the theory of psychosocial development. In this stage, the infant is completely dependent on its primary caregiver. It looks up to them for the fulfillment of its basic needs, security, and stability. The basic conflict encapsulates the question: Can the world be trusted?

The infant learns about the world and society through interactions with its parents. If the parents successfully provide the infant with security, comfort, affection, food, and warmth, the child will develop a sense of trust in the world around them and learn that others can be dependable. When it learns to trust the world, the infant acquires hope as a basic virtue. If the parents fail to show the infant that others can be trusted because they do not provide security, comfort, care, and affection, the infant will develop mistrust. It will learn that the world is inconsistent, unreliable, and unpredictable, which causes great anxiety and suspicion.

Stage Two: Autonomy versus Shame and Doubt (Between 18 Months and 3 Years)

In the second stage, the major crisis is about autonomy versus shame and doubt. During this stage, children start to develop more autonomy and a sense of independence, which is manifested in increased mobility and the discovery of new abilities, such as dressing up, picking up toys, etc. Children start to explore the world and their interests. Parents serve as a secure base from which toddlers can explore their newly found autonomy.

If parents successfully encourage a child's independence, the child will develop self-confidence and autonomy. The child will feel safe to explore the external environment and freely make choices. On the other hand, if parents are controlling and overly critical, the child will develop shame and doubt. The child might develop low self-esteem, which might prevent it from exploring the world freely and believing in its ability to lead an autonomous life.

According to Erikson, for the successful resolution of this stage, parents should aim for a delicate balance between encouraging children's exploration of their abilities and protecting them from constant failure.

Stage Three: Initiative versus Guilt (Between 3 and 6 Years)

The third stage of psychosocial development is the locomotor stage, in which children become active and begin to master their environment. They learn basic skills such as how to count, speak, plan, etc.

Children in this stage are energetic and lively. They start to understand that actions have a purpose. They play and interact with other children a lot. They learn how to control their environment with their decisions and actions. When a child takes the initiative for an action that does not cause the desired outcomes, this can lead to guilt—a new emotion for the child. The basic conflict during this stage is initiative versus guilt.

To encourage their children to develop a sense of initiative, parents should create a supportive environment in which kids are able to explore safely and freely. For example, in this stage, children may ask a lot of questions as their curiosity about the world grows. When parents respond to questions with annoyance, children might develop guilt, which can damage their curiosity and creativity.

If parents successfully find the balance between initiative and guilt, their children will learn they are allowed to make autonomous decisions, but they must also respect other people's rules. Children who successfully resolve this stage develop the virtue of purpose.

Stage Four: Industry versus Inferiority (Between 6 and 10 Years)

In the fourth stage of psychosocial development, children begin elementary school. They have interactions with their peers and teachers. Teachers and parents have increased expectations, and children start to develop confidence based on their abilities to fulfill those expectations. Children are expected to learn new skills and develop their individuality and moral code. They start to become responsible. They cooperate and share things with their peers, and they work on being "good" and try to do what's right. They learn to read, write, tell time, look at a calendar, develop a moral code, and become aware of cultural differences. Children start to develop interests such as sports, music, art, etc. This stage is critical for the development of healthy self-esteem and motivation.

In elementary school, children get feedback for their accomplishments and recognition from their parents and teachers. If they are encouraged and praised for their accomplishments and abilities, children will develop industry. They demonstrate this when they are responsible, finish tasks, and put in effort even if pleasure is delayed. If children are criticized, they may start to feel incapable and develop inferiority.

In this stage, parents and teachers play a vital role as they guide children in how to deal with failure, which is normal at this stage.

The social component is also developed in this stage. In school, children start to form social groups and compare themselves to their peers. Social interactions play a great role in the development of a person's self-confidence.

Stage Five: Identity versus Role Confusion (Between 12 and 18 Years)

This is the stage in which the transition from childhood to adulthood occurs. In this stage, adolescents explore their identity and their role in the world. The basic conflict is about identity versus role confusion, and the main existential question is: "Who am I, and what can I be?" Adolescents become concerned with how they appear to other people. They become curious about occupational, political, gender, religious, and sexual identities. For individuals to develop an identity, they need to be allowed to freely explore their values, motives, wishes, goals, and interests.

It's normal to experience role confusion at this stage. Adolescents may become confused about their role in the world, and they will experiment with different activities to sort out that confusion. According to Erikson, adolescents go through an identity crisis. The successful resolution of this crisis leads to the development of an integrated sense of self.

For the successful resolution of this stage, adolescents need to be given enough space and time to freely explore and find out by themselves who they truly are. Certain challenges might emerge, such as the establishment of boundaries and conflicts that arise with adults over expected societal roles. For example, parents might want their child to become a lawyer because they own a law firm, but their child might want to pursue a career in veterinary medicine. Parents must allow their children to develop their own identity. If a child is forced into a prechosen identity, this may cause rebellious behavior and a negative view of self.

If adolescents leave this stage with unresolved identity issues, they will become confused about their direction in life and their role in society. Consequently, they may develop a weak sense of self. An individual who successfully resolves this stage develops a strong identity and consistent values. Fidelity is the basic virtue acquired in this stage.

Stage Six: Intimacy versus Isolation (Between 20 and 45 Years)

The basic conflict of the sixth stage of psychosocial development is the formation of intimate connections versus isolation. According to Erikson, for individuals to be able to successfully form intimate relationships, the previous stage must be successfully resolved so individuals have a formed identity. An adult who is capable of close relationships can make sacrifices for others, is willing to be vulnerable with others, and has no issues with commitment. Someone who is not able to tolerate the loss of vulnerability and who fears commitment might avoid relationships and intimacy. This causes isolation and loneliness. The successful resolution of this stage results in meaningful relationships and the development of the virtue of love.

Stage Seven: Generativity versus Stagnation (Between 46 and 64 Years)

In this stage, adults aim to achieve generativity through contributions to the world and society. Since people in this stage are in midlife, their main concern is what they have contributed to society and what they will leave behind. Generativity is achieved when adults make an effort to contribute to positive societal changes that improve the lives of future generations. A sense of accomplishment is achieved if the individual has managed to raise a family or worked toward the improvement of society in some way. If a person has failed to work toward a meaningful goal, they will feel stagnation and emptiness.

In this stage, individuals are more focused on work. Productive and meaningful work is a great way to achieve a sense of purpose. Work can also bring a sense of community and belonging, especially if it improves the lives of other generations. Parenthood is another significant task during this part of life. When they teach values to children, adults gain a great sense of generativity. Other tasks that adults engage in include the creation and maintenance of a comfortable home, creative use of leisure time, the expression of love in various ways, etc.

The successful resolution of this stage leads to the development of the virtue of care. Adults who achieve this virtue feel they have left their mark on the world. Adults who have failed to achieve this virtue might feel a great disconnection with society and their community.

Stage Eight: Ego Integrity versus Despair (65 Years and Above)

This is the final stage of Erikson's stages of psychosocial development. In this stage, people reflect on the meaning of their lives. As they retire, productivity decreases, and they have more time for activities that don't involve work. People who feel like they have achieved their goals and have found a sense of purpose will develop ego integrity. They are content with how their lives turned out and feel a sense of satisfaction about their accomplishments.

Those who have successfully resolved the previous stages of development can more easily face any psychological conflicts that may occur in this stage. Individuals who develop ego integrity can look back on their lives and see them as successful and productive. Individuals who are dissatisfied with their lives and feel as if they have been unproductive or empty will develop despair. They might become depressed and fearful of death.

Chapter 2: Physiological Causes of Psychiatric Symptoms

Psychiatric mental health nurse practitioners should be aware that many medical conditions can present with psychiatric symptoms, and many mental illnesses may initially present with nonspecific somatic complaints. What makes matters even more complicated is that most medications can cause psychiatric side effects. Patients with chronic medical conditions may suffer from psychiatric diseases because of the debilitating nature of the medical disease that impairs their quality of life.

It's important to consider the frequent coexistence of psychiatric and medical conditions. Failure to recognize an underlying medical illness in patients who present with psychiatric symptoms delays proper treatment. This may cause the patient's condition to worsen. In this section, we provide an overview of the most common physiological causes of psychiatric symptoms.

Endocrinologic Disorders

Hypothyroidism

Hypothyroidism is caused by the primary failure of the thyroid gland, autoimmune thyroiditis (Hashimoto's), hypothalamic dysfunction, surgery or ablation of the thyroid gland, dysfunction of the pituitary gland, and lithium therapy. Patients present with fatigue, lethargy, weakness, irregularities in the menstrual cycle, dry skin, slow reaction time, cold intolerance, and bradycardia.

Hypothyroidism is a common cause of psychiatric symptoms such as depression, cognitive impairment, memory loss, irritability, and myxedema coma. Myxedema madness is a very rare severe psychosis caused by hypothyroidism. The cognitive impairment in hypothyroidism may occur as a consequence of depression in patients. Patients who present with depressive symptoms and cognitive impairment should be screened for hypothyroidism since the psychiatric symptoms are reversible if the underlying cause is treated.

Hyperthyroidism

Hyperthyroidism is caused by Graves' disease, toxic multinodular goiter, toxic adenoma, postpartum thyroiditis, and factitious hyperthyroidism. Hyperthyroidism presents with irritability, diaphoresis, palpitations, weight loss, dyspnea, tachycardia, excessive sweating, and fatigue. The most common psychiatric symptoms associated with hyperthyroidism are depression, anxiety, and cognitive impairment (memory loss, reduced productivity, and inattention). Hyperthyroidism can be diagnosed with thyroid function blood work. Psychiatric symptoms of hyperthyroidism resolve when the hyperthyroidism is treated with antithyroid medication, radioactive iodine, or surgery.

Cushing's syndrome

Cushing's syndrome most commonly occurs when there is increased secretion of cortisol by the adrenal gland or excessive exogenous glucocorticoid steroids are administered (e.g., in the treatment of chronic inflammatory diseases). Other causes of Cushing's syndrome include endogenous overproduction of glucocorticoid (e.g., a glucocorticoid-secreting tumor) or diseases of the pituitary gland. Since cortisol is normally secreted by the body in times of stress, elevated cortisol can be seen in psychiatric disorders.

Cortisol is elevated in major depressive disorder, panic disorder, anorexia nervosa, alcoholism, generalized anxiety disorder, and withdrawal from psychoactive substances. Cushing's syndrome presents with thin, atrophic skin, increased appetite, irregularities of the menstrual cycle, hypercholesterolemia, hypertriglyceridemia, glucose intolerance, hirsutism, fat redistribution, and striae. Psychiatric symptoms include dysphoria, irritability, insomnia, cognitive impairment (memory loss, inattention, problems with concentration), depressive and manic symptoms, and, in some cases, psychotic episodes. Psychiatric symptoms of Cushing's syndrome resolve when hypercortisolemia is normalized.

Primary Adrenal Insufficiency (Addison's Disease)

Adrenal insufficiency is characterized by reduced or diminished glucocorticoid and mineralocorticoid production. Addison's disease, also called primary adrenal insufficiency, is caused by the autoimmune destruction of the suprarenal glands. Adrenal insufficiency causes nonspecific symptoms that may overlap with other psychiatric diseases. Therefore, these patients are often misdiagnosed with major depressive disorder, dementia, or somatoform disorders. The clinical presentation consists of fatigue, diarrhea, weight loss, loss of appetite, and salt cravings. The diagnosis is made with laboratory measurement of serum adrenocorticotropic hormone (ACTH) and cortisol and diagnostic imaging of the pituitary and suprarenal glands. Psychiatric symptoms resolve once the hormone deficiency is corrected.

Metabolic Disorders

Vitamin Deficiency

Vitamin B1 (thiamine) deficiency causes Wernicke-Korsakoff syndrome. Wernicke encephalopathy is a syndrome characterized by a triad of ataxia, confusion, and oculomotor dysfunction. Korsakoff syndrome consists of anterograde and retrograde memory loss. Long-term memory is preserved in patients with Korsakoff syndrome. Alcohol use is another cause of Wernicke-Korsakoff syndrome.

The diagnosis is confirmed with laboratory measurements of serum thiamine. Patients with Wernicke encephalopathy can be treated with the replacement of thiamine, but some deficits might persist. Korsakoff syndrome is a chronic condition that requires long-term treatment and supportive care.

Vitamin B12 (cobalamin) is needed for DNA synthesis and proper neurological function. Vitamin B12 deficiency occurs due to malabsorption in conditions like pernicious anemia or when a person has a gastric/small bowel resection. Vitamin B12 deficiency is associated with many neuropsychiatric symptoms. Psychiatric symptoms include depression, anxiety, panic disorder, hallucinations, delusions, insomnia, mania, and psychosis. Neurologic symptoms include sensory polyneuropathy (impaired sense of vibration and proprioception), dysgeusia, urinary/fecal incontinence, cerebellar ataxia, cognitive impairment, spasticity, obtundation, and decreased visual acuity. The diagnosis is made with laboratory measurements of serum vitamin B12 levels. Symptoms are reversible with vitamin B12 replacement.

Calcium Disorders

Neuropsychiatric symptoms can occur as a result of elevated or decreased calcium levels in the blood. Hypocalcemia causes seizures, disorientation, confusion, emotional lability, delirium, anxiety, depression, and psychosis. Hypocalcemia can be a result of hypoparathyroidism, which occurs due to autoimmune destruction of the parathyroid glands, parathyroid or thyroid surgery, tumors, or disruption of the vascularity of the glands.

Correction of hypocalcemia with vitamin D and calcium supplementation will resolve the neuropsychiatric symptoms. Hypercalcemia causes confusion, weakness, lethargy, drowsiness, and depressive symptoms. Severe hypercalcemia may cause psychosis, stupor, coma, or death. Primary hyperparathyroidism and malignancy are the most common causes of hypercalcemia. Hypercalcemia may occur as a result of lithium therapy. Most symptoms resolve with treatment of the underlying cause, but some cognitive impairment may persist.

Wilson's Disease

Wilson's disease, also called hepatolenticular degeneration, is an autosomal recessive disorder that affects the hepatic transport of copper. This defect causes excessive copper deposition in organs, especially in the liver and the brain. Excessive copper deposition is responsible for organ injury. The onset of disease is insidious, and symptoms do not manifest before the age of six.

Wilson's disease causes both neurological and psychiatric symptoms. Neurologic symptoms include choreoathetosis, tremors, dystonia, ataxia, and cognitive impairment. Psychiatric symptoms include irritability, disinhibition, depression, aggression, and recklessness. The presence of a Kayser-Fleischer ring on an ophthalmologic slit-lamp examination raises the suspicion of Wilson's disease. The diagnosis can be made with 24-hour urine copper quantification. Proper diagnosis and treatment can enable afflicted individuals to have a normal life and prevent the onset of neuropsychiatric symptoms.

Autoimmune Disorders

Systemic Lupus Erythematosus

Systemic lupus erythematosus (SLE) is an autoimmune disorder caused by the presence of autoantibodies that injure several organs. The organs most commonly affected are the skin, kidneys, joints, and central nervous system. Symptoms of SLE include fatigue, fever, arthralgias, myalgias, weight loss, butterfly rash, photosensitivity, mucous ulcers, and Raynaud's phenomenon. Neuropsychiatric symptoms occur due to the presence of autoantibodies directed against neuronal membranes, and antibodies directed against NMDA receptors (N-methyl-D-aspartate).

Neurologic manifestations include cranial neuropathy, single or multiplex mononeuropathy, myelopathy, polyneuropathy, plexopathy, autonomic dysfunction, aseptic meningitis, cerebrovascular disease, chorea, seizures, Guillain-Barré syndrome. Psychiatric manifestations include depression, mood disorders, anxiety disorders, psychosis, and cognitive decline (memory impairment, learning difficulties). The diagnosis is confirmed with laboratory measurement of high-titer antinuclear antibodies (ANA) and other specific autoantibodies like anti-dsDNA and anti-Smith antibodies.

Treatment consists of corticosteroids and immunosuppressive medications like azathioprine and cyclophosphamide. Lupus psychosis is treated with antipsychotics. In certain cases, steroid treatment induces psychiatric symptoms. Distinguishing steroid psychosis from psychosis caused by CNS lupus is a difficult diagnostic dilemma that requires close collaboration between psychiatrists and rheumatologists.

Gastrointestinal Disorders

Esophageal dysmotility

Esophageal dysmotility can be a cause of noncardiac chest pain that leads many patients to seek psychiatric consultation. Certain psychiatric illnesses have been linked to esophageal dysmotility. Patients with esophageal dysmotility most commonly suffer from major depressive disorder (up to 52%), generalized anxiety disorder (36%), somatization disorder (20%), and substance-use disorders (20%).

The treatment consists of smooth muscle relaxants. Antidepressants and behavioral therapies improve the patient's subjective complaints and psychological well-being.

Irritable Bowel Syndrome

Irritable bowel syndrome is associated with stress due to increased sensitivity of the enteric nervous system to stress. Emotional stress causes increased sympathetic nervous system activity, which causes inhibition of gastric motility. The symptoms of irritable bowel syndrome include abdominal pain relieved by defecation, bloating, passage of mucus, and altered stool frequency, form, and passage.

Psychiatric disorders are frequently found in patients who suffer from IBS. The most common ones are panic disorder (26%), social phobia (26%), generalized anxiety disorder (26%), and major depressive disorder (23%). Tricyclic antidepressants are beneficial for patients who suffer from diarrhea and IBS due to their anticholinergic effect. Most patients with IBS improve with low-dose antidepressants or antianxiety medications, even those without a psychiatric disorder.

Gastroesophageal Reflux and Peptic Ulcer Disease

Gastroesophageal reflux and peptic ulcer disease cause epigastric noncardiac chest pain one to three hours after a meal. Major risk factors of peptic ulcer disease are infection with *Helicobacter Pylori* and excessive use of nonsteroidal anti-inflammatory drugs. Many patients who have non-ulcer dyspepsia suffer from a psychiatric comorbidity. Depression is the most common psychiatric disorder in patients with gastroesophageal reflux disease.

Respiratory Disorders

Chronic Obstructive Pulmonary Disease (COPD)

Chronic obstructive pulmonary disease (COPD) is a disease characterized by the slow, progressive obstruction of airways, which presents with dyspnea, cough, and excessive sputum production. COPD affects middle-aged and older adults and chronic smokers. On physical examination, patients present with lung overinflation, use of accessory muscles that help with respiration, wheezing on auscultation, and diminished breath sounds.

Psychiatric symptoms in patients with COPD may be due to chronic hypoxia or treatment with corticosteroid medications. Chronic hypoxia causes cognitive deficits and mood disorders. Patients may present with depression, mood lability, or delirium. Increased carbon dioxide levels in the blood can cause panic attacks. Benzodiazepines are not useful for panic attacks in patients with COPD because they suppress respiratory function. Neuroleptics should be used with caution in patients with COPD due to potential respiratory side effects.

Obstructive Sleep Apnea (OSA)

Obstructive sleep apnea (OSA) is an obstruction of the upper airways that causes the complete cessation of airflow during sleep. The obstructive episodes usually last for 10 seconds or more, and they occur most commonly during REM sleep. Apneic episodes can happen in any individual, but their increase in frequency can cause excessive daytime sleepiness and decreased sleep quality.

Obstructive sleep apnea is associated with many psychiatric symptoms, such as neurocognitive impairment, impaired focus, depression, anxiety, insomnia, personality changes, and irritability. Sleep apnea can also cause marital problems. Partners may begin to sleep in another room due to the inability to tolerate loud snoring and restlessness.

Risk factors for sleep apnea include obesity, use of sedating drugs, and alcohol-use disorder. Patients who report chronic fatigue, excessive daytime sleepiness, depression, poor motivation, and impaired concentration can be screened for sleep apnea during the psychiatric interview. Continuous positive airway pressure (CPAP) is an effective treatment for sleep apnea that can resolve most symptoms.

Cardiovascular Disorders

Type A and type D personality

An understanding of a patient's personality can potentially predict their cardiovascular morbidity and mortality. For instance, type A personality increases the risk of myocardial infarction. People with type A personalities are ambitious, competitive, impatient, aggressive, alert, have a high potential for anger, get easily irritated, and suffer from muscle tension. They can describe themselves as "workaholics," and they pride themselves on being resistant to emotional "weakness." These patients need to control their environment. Modification of the behavior of a patient with a type A personality who has had a previous myocardial infarction can prevent future infarctions.

A type D personality is characterized by the avoidance of social interactions and the inhibition of negative emotions. People with type D personalities have an increased risk of cardiovascular morbidity and mortality, but the association between type D personality and increased cortisol needs more research to be confirmed. The association between type D personality and cardiac risk needs more research to be confirmed.

Chapter 3: Psychiatric Disorders

Schizophrenia Spectrum

Psychotic disorders are severely debilitating psychiatric disorders with different etiologies characterized by the inability of the patient to recognize reality. Schizophrenia is a severe mental disorder that causes significant, long-lasting impairments and disability. Men are more affected by schizophrenia than women. They usually have an earlier onset of the disease, more negative symptoms, and poorer prognosis. Women tend to have more dysphoria, paranoid delusions, and hallucinations compared to men.

The underlying cause is not known, but various theories implicate a genetic component, neurodevelopmental abnormalities, neurobiological defects, and others. Schizophrenia causes impairments in perception, cognition, emotion, behavior, eye movement, and socialization. Symptoms of most psychiatric disorders can be seen in schizophrenia. Therefore, there is no sign or symptom that is pathognomonic for this disorder.

Perception abnormalities of schizophrenia include delusions and hallucinations. Delusions can be persecutory, grandiose, erotomanic, jealous, religious, and somatic. Patients may believe they are being controlled by an outside entity or that they can control the outside world. Hallucinations are most commonly auditory, but all five senses may be affected. Tactile, gustatory, and olfactory hallucinations are very rare, and their presence may point toward an underlying neurological or medical cause of psychosis. Patients hear voices that may insult or threaten them. The voices may have conversations between themselves.

Patients with schizophrenia have disorganized thinking characterized by an inability to organize and interpret information. Both the process and content of their thoughts are affected. This can be reflected in the patient's speech, which is often referred to as "word salad" due to its incomprehensibility.

Affective symptoms of schizophrenia may range from anhedonia to extreme rage, depression, and anxiety. Patients often have a flat or blunted affect. Behavior is unusual, and it may range from silliness to unpredictable anger.

Schizophrenia symptoms can be divided into three categories: positive, negative, and cognitive symptoms. Positive symptoms include hallucinations, delusions, and disorganized thinking. Positive symptoms are seen during an acute psychotic episode. Negative symptoms refer to the absence of normal behavior, and they include blunted affect, absence of motivation, pleasure, attention, and thought.

Cognitive impairment affects attention, episodic memory, working memory, and executive function. Cognitive symptoms cause a lot of the disability associated with schizophrenia.

Mood Disorders

Bipolar Disorders

Bipolar disorders include bipolar disorder type I and II and cyclothymia. Bipolar disorders are characterized by manic, hypomanic, and depressive episodes. The hallmark of a manic episode is an increased, uninhibited, or irritable mood that lasts for at least one week. The patient in a manic episode is very talkative, amusing, euphoric, and speaks with a sense of urgency, which is referred to as pressured speech.

The patient may exhibit risky behaviors, such as unrestrained shopping sprees, unsafe promiscuous behavior, and excessive substance use. Patients have a decreased need for sleep and are hyperactive. They have impaired judgment and may become combative or threatening. Patients in a manic episode frequently require hospitalization and may suffer from psychotic symptoms such as delusions and hallucinations.

Hypomania is similar to mania. However, it has a shorter duration, less severe clinical presentation, and does not require hospitalization. Depressive episodes in bipolar disorders are similar to those seen in major depressive disorders. Bipolar I patients have one or more manic or mixed episodes. Bipolar II patients have one or more depressive episodes and at least one hypomanic episode. Cyclothymia is a type of disorder that is described as a less severe form of bipolar disorder.

Depressive Disorders

The hallmark of a depressed mood is the loss of pleasure or interest. Major depressive disorder (MDD) is a common psychiatric disorder that has multifactorial etiologies, which include biochemical, environmental, and genetic theories. MDD affects 5% of adults in the US and is the leading cause of disability. The clinical presentation of MDD consists of a loss of pleasure (anhedonia), a decrease or increase in weight or appetite, sleep, or activity, a decrease in energy, psychomotor retardation, dysphoria, impaired concentration, depressive thoughts filled with worthlessness and guilt, and suicidal ideation.

To diagnose MDD, the symptoms must be present for at least two weeks. Psychotic symptoms may occur during a depressive episode. This is referred to as depression with psychotic features. Dysthymic disorder is a less severe form of major depressive disorder. The hallmark of dysthymia is a continuous depressive mood that begins in childhood or adolescence. Major depressive disorder causes psychosocial consequences such as impaired social, occupational, and relational functioning.

Neurocognitive Disorders

Cognitive disorders are characterized by a disruption in one or more of the following domains: language, memory, judgment, orientation, interpersonal relationships, problem-solving, and praxis (performing functions). They are often accompanied by abnormal behavior. Neurocognitive disorders are caused by a medical or neurological condition that manifests as psychiatric and/or neurologic symptomatology and changes in cognition. The deficit in cognition is a major change from the patient's previous level of functioning. These disorders most commonly affect older adults, but they may occur at any age. Delirium and dementia are the most common neurocognitive disorders.

Delirium

Delirium is a syndrome with an acute onset characterized by a short-term decline in consciousness and cognition. Delirium may occur due to a general medical condition, substance use, multiple physical health etiologies, and others (e.g., sleep deprivation, medications, etc.). Older adults are most affected by delirium. The disturbance of consciousness usually develops over hours to a few days, and it fluctuates throughout the day.

Psychiatric symptoms of delirium include abnormalities of mood, perception, and behavior. Patients may present with agitation, restlessness, apathy, or lethargy. They may present with nonspecific neurological signs such as tremors, myoclonus, asterixis, nystagmus, and others. Due to impaired consciousness, patients are at risk of accidental injury. Delirium resolves after treatment of the underlying cause.

Dementia

Dementia, also referred to as a major neurocognitive disorder, is a condition characterized by a progressive decline of cognitive abilities, which causes major impairment in the patient's occupational and social functioning. Dementia can be classified into multiple types based on its etiology: Lewy body dementia, vascular dementia, Alzheimer's disease, frontotemporal dementia, traumatic brain injury (TBI), HIV, Parkinson's disease, prion disease, Huntington's disease, and other medical or neurological disorders.

To make a diagnosis of dementia, the clinician relies on information that is gathered from the clinical and mental status exam, and information from the patient's close family or friends, as well as neuroimaging and laboratory tests. Patients present with cognitive impairment in attention, language, learning, memory, executive function, perception, movement, and social cognition. The clinical presentation may vary in different types of dementia. Patients may present with personality changes such as accentuation of previous personality traits, introversion, and increased hostility and irritability. Hostility may be pronounced in patients who suffer from paranoid delusions.

Hallucinations are present in 20 to 30% of patients with dementia, and delusions are present in 30 to 40%. Mood disorders such as depression and anxiety are present in 40 to 50% of patients. Treatment of dementia is supportive, preventive, and pharmacological.

Personality Disorders

Personality disorders are characterized by long-lasting maladaptive behaviors and abnormal relating to oneself and others that cause impairments in multiple areas of functioning. Patients with personality disorders are often unaware of their maladaptive behavior, and they try to change the external environment instead of themselves. Patients with personality disorders often reject treatment. They are often diagnosed after they complain of a comorbid disorder that has occurred as a consequence of their personality disorder. According to the DSM-V, specific personality disorders are divided into clusters A, B, and C.

Cluster A: Odd and Eccentric

This category is comprised of paranoid personality disorder, schizoid personality disorder, and schizotypal personality disorder. Patients with paranoid personality disorders are excessively suspicious of others. They are distrustful and may interpret other's intentions as threatening, deceptive, or hostile. They frequently have trouble in interpersonal relationships due to pathological jealousy.

Patients with schizoid personality disorder are uninterested and detached from interpersonal relationships. They have few or no friends or acquaintances and spend most of their time alone. They appear quiet, unsociable, emotionally constricted, reserved, aloof, and self-absorbed.

The hallmark of schizotypal personality disorder is difficulty maintaining interpersonal relationships and eccentric behavior. These patients have disturbed thought and communication with the absence of the actual thought disorder. These patients are often isolated and unsociable. They frequently have superstitious beliefs and may believe they possess special powers. They are at risk of developing psychotic symptoms when they are under stress.

Cluster B: Dramatic

This category is comprised of antisocial personality disorder, borderline personality disorder, histrionic personality disorder, and narcissistic personality disorder. Patients with antisocial personality disorder are characterized by a pervasive disrespect for other people's rights. These patients are frequently diagnosed with conduct disorder in their childhood or have evidence of behaviors that point towards conduct disorder. At first, these patients may appear charming or manipulative. They may lie, abuse others, or commit crimes. They have no remorse for their actions, as if they have no conscience.

BPD is characterized by chaotic, intense interpersonal relationships, intense fear of abandonment and frantic efforts to avoid it, impulsive behavior, affective instability, chronic sense of emptiness, identity disturbance, black-and-white thinking (often called splitting), chronic or recurrent suicidality, and dissociative symptoms. Patients with BPD are at risk of psychosis under stress.

Histrionic personality disorder is characterized by a high need for attention manifested by attention-seeking behaviors such as seductiveness, flirtatiousness, flamboyancy, exaggerated speech, and promiscuity. These patients are uncomfortable when they are not the center of attention, and they manifest temper tantrums.

The hallmark of narcissistic personality disorder is an exaggerated sense of self-importance and grandiosity. These patients lack empathy for others and may exhibit exploitative behaviors and arrogance. They feel special or unique and expect special treatment and validation from others.

Cluster C: Anxious

Patients with avoidant personality disorder lack confidence and are very sensitive to rejection. They are afraid of being disliked, and therefore, they avoid relationships because of shame. They are very inhibited in relationships and fear criticism.

Patients with dependent personality disorder are submissive and dependent on others. They are unable to make decisions by themselves and usually avoid responsibility or leadership. They need to be attached to another person, and they quickly seek out new relationships when a previous one ends.

Obsessive-compulsive personality disorder (OCPD) is characterized by a preoccupation with order, rules, and regulations. These patients are perfectionistic and have high expectations of others. Their personality is constricted, and they have problems in interpersonal relationships.

Anxiety Disorders

Anxiety disorders are the most common mental health disorders in the USA. They are a major cause of social and occupational dysfunction. Anxiety presents with many symptoms, both physical and psychological. Physical symptoms are most commonly due to overactivation of the sympathetic branch of the autonomic nervous system. They include palpitations, tachycardia, headaches, excessive sweating, chest tightness, and gastrointestinal discomfort. Motor symptoms such as restlessness may be present as well.

In severe anxiety, patients may have disorganized or negative thinking. Patients catastrophize and ruminate on potential dangers. Patients who have panic attacks may think they're dying or having a heart attack. Patients with anxiety disorders have a higher risk of suicide compared to people without mental disorders.

Anxiety disorders include panic disorder (with or without agoraphobia), specific phobia (fear of blood, injury, injections, situational phobia, animals, and others), social anxiety disorder, agoraphobia, and generalized anxiety disorder.

Panic attacks are intense, abrupt, unpredictable anxiety attacks that may last from minutes to hours and are accompanied by physical manifestations (cardiopulmonary, gastrointestinal, neurologic, psychiatric) and a feeling of impending doom. Patients exhibit avoidance behavior. They try to avoid triggers that may induce another attack, and they have anticipatory anxiety in between attacks (they are afraid of another attack).

Agoraphobia is characterized by a fear of being in situations or places that might be difficult to escape. It causes occupational and social dysfunction since patients with agoraphobia may find it very difficult to leave their homes. It may occur with or without a panic disorder.

Specific phobia is characterized by a fear of a specific object or situation that causes avoidance behaviors (avoiding the specific object or situation) and severe distress.

Social anxiety disorder is characterized by anxiety in social situations due to fears of being judged. Patients with this disorder tend to avoid social situations, which causes psychosocial distress and impairment.

Generalized anxiety disorder (GAD) is characterized by anxiety about most situations and activities. For the diagnosis of GAD to be made, the symptoms must be present for at least six months. GAD is frequently accompanied by somatic symptoms such as insomnia, muscle tension, headaches, and irritability.

Chapter 4: Coping and Defense Mechanisms

Coping mechanisms are thoughts and behaviors that can be used to overcome or manage stressful situations. When a person is going through a stressful situation, the behavior they use to deal with stress is called their coping style. One way of coping is to consciously seek support from others. Another way is through conscious cognitive strategies. Defense mechanisms are involuntary, subconscious, adaptive coping mechanisms that can alter one's perception of reality. Using defense mechanisms can reduce feelings of anxiety, depression, and distress.

Coping can be divided into problem-focused, emotion-focused, meaning-focused, and social coping. Problem-focused coping is characterized by active efforts to cope by use of information support, planning, and positive reframing. The strategies that the individual uses aim to change the situation. An example of problem-focused coping is when an individual reads about the topic and creates strategies to overcome the situation based on available information.

Emotion-focused coping is characterized by acts that reduce negative emotions. It consists of venting, acceptance of the situation, spirituality or religion, and self-blame. Examples of emotion-focused coping are conversations with friends about the situation, jokes, prayer, or meditation.

Meaning-focused coping is characterized by cognitively seeking a higher meaning from the situation that might improve one's life in the future. Social coping is characterized by seeking help from one's community.

Some individuals use maladaptive coping, such as avoidant coping, suppression of emotions, and behavioral disengagement. Avoidant coping includes self-destruction, use of substances and alcohol, and denial. Maladaptive coping mechanisms are associated with decreased mental health and a higher incidence of psychopathology.

Coping can also be divided into proactive or reactive. People who are proactive take measures to prevent a stressful situation from occurring, and they build resilience against future stressful events. They are more adaptive to a stable environment. These people prefer routines and structure. Reactive people are better at neutralizing stressful situations. Coping scales can be used to determine an individual's coping style. Some examples include the COPE scale (Coping Orientation to Problems Experienced), Coping Inventory for Stressful Situations, and Coping Response Inventory.

Defense Mechanisms

Defense mechanisms are unconscious psychological strategies that an individual uses when faced with a situation that can cause anxiety, depression, or distress. They can be necessary when a person needs to adjust to a reality that cannot be immediately integrated. However, excessive use of defense mechanisms is associated with psychopathology and neuroses like anxiety, phobias, and obsessions.

Primitive Defense Mechanisms

Denial

Denial is a defense mechanism that occurs when an individual denies facts of objective reality that may be too much to handle. People who are in denial dismiss external reality. For example, denial may be used by individuals who have serious substance abuse problems but refuse to admit it to themselves and others.

Acting out

Acting out is characterized by behaviors that distract from the stressful situation. Acting out can be seen in antisocial personality disorder, oppositional defiant disorder, or conduct disorder.

Repression

Repression is characterized by blocking undesirable and uncomfortable feelings, ideas, memories, or impulses. This defense mechanism is seen in people who have survived a traumatic event but have no conscious recollection of it, even though they did not lose consciousness when it occurred.

Projection

If an individual has problems accepting their thoughts, traits, feelings, and motives, they might project them onto other people. This defense mechanism serves to protect the person's self-concept. By projecting unwanted traits onto other people, they deny the existence of these traits in themselves. For example, if a person cheats in a relationship, they might project by being excessively jealous or suspicious of their partner's fidelity.

Regression

When individuals are faced with a stressful situation, they might revert to an earlier stage of development, like a kind of psychological time-travel. For example, someone who has lost a pet might start to display behavior seen in children. They might scream, kick, bite, wet the bed, or throw temper tantrums. Another example of regression: A patient going through a divorce starts to suck his thumb. He says he hasn't done that in years, but it used to be a comforting behavior.

Conversion

Conversion is the transformation of intolerable psychiatric symptoms into physical symptoms that cannot be explained by an underlying medical cause or injury. This defense mechanism might cause conversion disorder. An example of conversion: A young female patient prepares to move to another country for the first time in her life.

She says she is ready and not afraid of the big change. She reports that in the last month, she has had trouble breathing and suffers from headaches almost every day.

Introjection

Introjection involves subsuming someone else's personality traits into one's own personality. Behaviors, thoughts, and characteristics of other people are internalized in the person's self-concept. Freud believed that superegos are developed through introjection. An example of introjection: A patient grew up with a very critical father. The patient has internalized her father's criticism and now has issues with self-esteem. She puts herself down and has trouble accepting good things in her life. As a consequence of low self-esteem, the patient has developed MDD.

Identification with the Aggressor

This defense mechanism occurs when a victim adopts the behavior of an aggressor in an attempt to avoid abuse and induce feelings of empathy. When victims identify with their aggressor, they adopt the aggressor's negative traits. Stockholm syndrome is an extreme type of identification with the aggressor. In Stockholm syndrome, victims who are held hostage develop an emotional bond with their captors. The case of Patty Hearst is an example of Stockholm syndrome. She was kidnapped by the Symbionese Liberation Army, which abused and brainwashed her. She changed her name, joined the group, and participated in bank robberies.

Splitting

Splitting is a failure to recognize the positive and negative characteristics of a person or situation due to conflicting emotions. This results in black-or-white thinking. Splitting is a normal way of thinking during childhood. Children might have polarized views on the world and others, but as they get older, they start to integrate negative and positive views. If a child is exposed to many negative situations, the integration might be interrupted and cause poor self-development.

Splitting is commonly seen in BPD. People with BPD might idealize someone and see them as a perfect being, and the moment that person does something perceived as wrong or hurtful, they might devalue them and see them as someone who has only negative characteristics. The idealization-devaluation cycle largely depends on how much an individual's emotional needs are met. Splitting can cause chaotic interpersonal relationships.

Undoing

Undoing occurs when someone ruminates on the past by reimagining a different outcome to protect themselves from negative feelings. An example of undoing: A couple had an argument that led to their breakup. One of the partners starts to regret the separation, and he keeps reimagining an alternative scenario in which they stay together.

Dissociation

Dissociation occurs when people detach from themselves (depersonalization) or their environment (derealization) to cope with stress. Dissociation also includes a break in memory formation as a protection against high stress. This may cause amnesia or a fragmented sense of self. When someone dissociates, they are protecting themselves from intense emotions by not integrating the stressful event into their consciousness. An example of dissociation is excessive daydreaming.

Higher-level Defense Mechanisms

Anticipation

This is a defense mechanism that consists of efforts to solve a problem before it arises. People who use anticipation can predict future problematic events and act accordingly. An example of anticipation would be a student who, to prepare for a difficult exam, practices the hardest questions.

Compensation

Compensation occurs when someone attempts to make up for flaws in one area of their life by devoting more attention and effort to another area. If the compensation is excessive, it's called overcompensation. An example of overcompensation is a young male who feels inadequate because of his low muscle tone. He starts to lift weights and drink protein shakes. He becomes very muscular and overcompensates for what he perceives to be a physical flaw.

Displacement

Displacement is the transfer of an emotional impulse from one entity to another. The person displaces a strong emotion on a more suitable target. An example of displacement: Oliver is angry because his boss makes him work overtime. He is unable to protest against his boss. When he comes home, he yells at his son for no reason. Oliver displaces his anger toward his boss, who is an unacceptable target, onto his son.

Humor

When a person uses humor as a defense mechanism, this is a way of pairing negative emotions with comedy to lessen their impact.

Intellectualization

Someone who uses intellectualization as a defense mechanism will start to overanalyze and ruminate about the situation, gather facts, and make conclusions. Intellectualization puts a distance between a person and powerful emotions. An example of intellectualization is when someone discovers they have an illness. Instead of showing emotions, they may start to research everything about the disease.

Rationalization

Rationalization occurs when someone tries to justify uncomfortable feelings, thoughts, or behaviors through logical or rational explanations. An example of rationalization: Fred failed to show up for a job interview on time, and he did not get the job because of this. To avoid disappointment, he says, "I didn't want the job anyway!"

Reaction Formation

Reaction formation occurs when someone behaves in the opposite way of what they're truly feeling. The opposite behaviors the person exhibits are conscious ways to try to overcompensate for the unconscious unacceptable or uncomfortable feelings.

An example of reaction formation: Beth has a new roommate. She dislikes her roommate's habits, and over time, she starts to resent her. Beth is uncomfortable with this resentment since she will have to continue to live with her roommate for the next year. Beth is extremely kind to her roommate and showers her with gifts, even though she deeply dislikes her.

Sublimation

Sublimation is a defense mechanism that is similar to displacement. Sublimation occurs when uncomfortable emotions are transformed into socially acceptable behaviors. An example of sublimation is when someone who has uncontrollable anger issues starts a high-intensity sport.

Suppression

Suppression is similar to repression, but while repression is unconscious, suppression is a process in which a person consciously chooses to suppress certain uncomfortable or unacceptable thoughts and feelings. An example of suppression is someone who has survived a very traumatic event and continues to have intrusive thoughts about it during the workday. They choose to consciously suppress their intrusive thoughts so they can focus on the task at hand.

Professional Intervention and Monitoring

Educating patients and their families about healthy coping skills can cause a significant improvement in the way they manage their illness and other problems in their personal lives. When patients are enabled to use healthier coping skills, this increases their responsibility for their health. It's important to identify patients who have maladaptive coping styles since these patients are more likely to be noncompliant with their treatment and engage in risky behaviors. Psychodynamic therapy can help patients become aware of their coping and defense mechanisms. Identifying unconscious processes can lead to a better outcome in many psychiatric disorders, such as depression, eating disorders, anxiety disorders, and personality disorders.

Chapter 5: Assessment Tools and Techniques

The Psychiatric Interview

The main parts of the psychiatric interview are the patient history and mental status examination. The patient history consists of subjective information obtained from patients or families/caretakers during the interview. The mental status examination is an objective tool similar to the physical examination.

The initial interview begins with the collection of basic information about the patient (name, age, marital status, sex, race or ethnicity, and occupation). The second part of the interview assesses the source and reliability of the information. This is needed to know where the information comes from and its reliability. The third part is the chief complaint, which consists of the main symptom the patient is bothered by. This is written in the patient's own words. An example is "I feel very anxious."

History of Present Illness

The history of the present illness is a chronological description of the course of symptoms. This section can begin with an open-ended question such as "What brought you here today?" In some cases, the clinician will have to guide the patient.

Information that should be obtained includes the type of symptoms, how long they have been present, the severity of symptoms, fluctuations in the severity or nature, presence or absence of stressors (situations at home, school, work, presence of medical disease, difficulties in interpersonal relationships), and factors that alleviate or worsen symptoms (support, coping skills, behaviors, medications).

Other important information that should be asked is why the patient chose to seek help now and the situation in which the illness began. A psychiatric review of systems should be included to identify potential comorbid disorders. The review is divided into several categories, such as anxiety, psychosis, mood, and others (including symptoms of ADHD, eating disorders).

Past Psychiatric History

The psychiatric mental health nurse practitioner should gather detailed information about previous psychiatric illnesses, their evolution over the patient's life, prior episodes of the current illness, and the frequency and severity of previous episodes. Detailed information about past treatment should also be included: inpatient treatment (voluntary or involuntary hospitalization), outpatient treatment (psychotherapy, day treatment, partial hospitalization), medications, electroconvulsive therapy, and other treatment modalities.

Substance Use, Abuse, and Addictions

Questions about substance use, abuse, and addictions should be asked in a nonjudgmental manner so the psychiatric mental health nurse practitioner can obtain accurate information. The history should include what type of substances have been used, the route of use, frequency and amount of use, tolerance, withdrawal symptoms, need for increasing amounts, impact on social interactions, schoolwork, and legal consequences. The CAGE or RAPS4 are brief standardized questionnaires that can be used to identify alcohol use disorders.

Other information that should be obtained includes periods of sobriety and settings in which they occurred, history of previous treatment (detoxification, rehabilitation, outpatient treatment, self-help groups, or group therapy), current substance abuse or dependence, possible behavioral addictions, tobacco and caffeine use, and eating behaviors.

Past Medical History

This section should include the presence of any medical conditions, surgical history, and treatment. A medical condition can worsen the symptoms of a psychiatric illness, such as when a patient with anxiety is diagnosed with cancer. A medical condition can also mimic a psychiatric illness (hypothyroidism mimics MDD), or it can be precipitated by the treatment of a psychiatric illness (metabolic syndrome caused by second-generation antipsychotics). It is very important to note the use of any nonpsychiatric medications and other treatments, including herbs since they can affect the metabolism of psychiatric medications.

Family History

Many mental illnesses have a genetic component in their etiology. Therefore, a detailed family history is an important part of the psychiatric interview. Family history can provide information about risk factors for certain illnesses. For example, a family history of suicide may increase the risk of suicidality in the patient.

Developmental and Social History

This section contains information about the patient's life, development, and psychosocial stressors. The childhood history consists of information about the patient's home environment and childhood friendships. School history contains information on the patient's academic success or difficulties, learning disorders, extracurricular activities, and behavioral history. Work history contains information about the types of jobs the patient has worked, how frequently the patient changes jobs, work performance, and relationships with authorities and coworkers. Relationships and marriage history reflect the patient's ability to develop and maintain interpersonal relationships. Other important information includes legal history, hobbies and interests, cultural and religious beliefs, and others.

Mental Status Examination

The mental status examination (MSE) is an objective tool that gathers information about areas of mental function and signs and symptoms of psychiatric disease. The MSE begins from the moment the patient enters the room in the first interaction. The information is gathered from observation. It reveals information about the current mental state of the patient, which can be used to monitor progress over time.

Appearance and Behavior

In this section, patients' general appearance is assessed. How do they look and behave? Does a patient look like his age? What is someone wearing, and is it appropriate? Does an individual look like he takes care of his hygiene and grooming? Are there any distinguishing features, such as tattoos, scars, and disfigurations? Is the patient cooperative, uncooperative, agitated, disinhibited, disinterested, etc.?

Motor Activity

Assessment of motor activity can provide valuable diagnostic information. It can give clues about the presence of depression, mania, attention-deficiency hyperactivity disorder, anxiety, adverse reactions from medications (parkinsonism due to antipsychotic medications), and others. Motor activity is described as bradykinesia (slow) or hyperactivity (agitated). The psychiatric mental health nurse practitioner should note the presence or absence of tics, jitteriness, restlessness, tongue protrusions, lip-smacking, tremors, unusual or sustained postures, and freedom of movement.

Speech

The elements of speech that should be evaluated include fluency, speed, amount, volume, and tone. Fluency is related to the command the patient has in their mother tongue. Speed is an important element since it can provide diagnostic clues. Slow speech is associated with depression. Rapid and pressured speech can be seen in mania or hypomania. The amount of speech can be increased (mania, hypomania, ADHD) or decreased (depression, psychosis, thought blocking). Tone and volume of speech can be described as dysphoric, irritable, loud, anxious, quiet, timid, childlike, or angry.

Mood

Mood can be defined as the internal emotional experience of a patient. Since it is a subjective state, the patient's words should be used when describing mood. Mood can be described as sad, happy, angry, guilty, depressed, anxious, etc.

Affect

Affect is the external expression of the patient's mood or what it appears to be to the person (doctor or nurse) who examines the patient. Affect can be described in terms of quality, quantity, appropriateness, range, and congruence. The quality can be described as euthymic, happy, irritable, dysphoric, angry, tearful, agitated, blunted, and flat.

Quantity measures the intensity of affect and describes it as mild or severe. The emotional range can be described as normal, broad (full), or constricted. Severely constricted affect is called flat affect, and it is often seen in patients with schizophrenia. Appropriateness describes how appropriate the affect is according to the setting. Congruency refers to the compatibility of the affect with the patient's mood or thought content. For example, a patient who reports sadness but laughs is said to have an incongruent affect.

Thought Content

Thought content is the type of thoughts in the patient's mind. Obsessive thoughts are repetitive thoughts that are unwelcome and resisted by the patient. Compulsions are behaviors that are repetitive and ritualized. Patients perform compulsions in order to decrease anxiety or distress or to avoid a certain outcome. Delusions are false, fixed beliefs that can be bizarre (out of the realm of possibility) or non-bizarre (not out of the realm of possibility but not true). Delusions can be categorized as grandiose, jealous, persecutory, somatic, and erotomanic. The patient must be asked about suicidal or homicidal thoughts, including their intent, sense of ideation, potential plan, and preparation.

Thought Process

The thought process refers to the formulation, organization, and expression of thoughts. It does not take into account the content. The normal thought process is goal-directed, linear, and organized. Examples of abnormal thought processes include flight of ideas, circumstantiality, clang association, thought blocking, tangential thoughts, loose thoughts or associations, perseveration, and derailment. For example, a patient with a flight of ideas rapidly moves from one topic to another. The ideas are logically connected, but they are hard to keep up with. In loose associations, there is rapid movement from one thought to another, but the thoughts are not connected logically. Perseveration refers to the failure of the patient to move on to other topics despite the clinician's attempt to change the fixated topic of conversation.

Perceptual Disturbances

Perceptual disturbances are illusions, hallucinations, depersonalization, and derealization. Hallucinations occur when there is a perception without an external stimulus. Hallucinations can be auditory, visual, tactile, gustatory, and olfactory. Derealization is a feeling that the environment is changed or unreal. Depersonalization is a feeling that something within oneself is not real.

Cognition

Cognition consists of alertness, orientation, concentration, memory, calculation, knowledge, abstract reasoning, insight, and judgment. Alertness is tested through observations of patients and their functioning. Orientation can be tested by asking patients general questions like name, location, etc. To test concentration, the patient can be asked to count backward by seven from 100. To test memory, the patient can be asked to repeat words or numbers (short-term memory), or questions can be asked about their childhood. To test calculations, the patient can be asked to solve simple math problems. Fund of knowledge depends on culture and educational background. To test it, the patient can be asked general questions. To test abstract reasoning, the patient can be asked to interpret proverbs or identify similarities between objects.

Insight refers to the patient's understanding of the presence of his psychiatric illness. Insight can be absent, partial, or full. A patient who is psychotic may say, "I am aware that there are no aliens coming to get me, but I can hear their voices even though I know they're not there." This patient has insight even though he suffers from a severe psychiatric disease. It's important to distinguish judgment from insight. Judgment is the patient's ability to make good or bad decisions and act on them.

Suicide Risk Assessment

The strongest risk factors for suicidality are previous suicide attempts and the presence of a psychiatric disorder. A psychiatric mental health nurse practitioner can use screening instruments to identify patients who are at risk. The Emergency Department Safety Assessment and Follow-up Evaluation (ED-SAFE) is a type of instrument used universally on every patient who presents to the emergency department (ED) regardless of the chief complaint. Other instruments that can be used include the C-SSRS and the SAFE-T Pocket Card.

Screening instruments are combined with clinical assessment of risk. A suicide assessment is done on all patients. It includes prior history, family history of suicide attempts, and completed suicides. The patient should be asked about current ideation, plan, and intent. Prior attempts should be assessed for potential triggers and their lethality risk. It is necessary to ask the patient about current thoughts of suicide and intent. A patient who has thoughts of suicide without intent to act on them has "suicidal ideation without intent." The nurse should ask the patient about the type of plan and assess whether the person has access to means that would enable them to complete the plan. Ask the patient what has previously prevented them from ending their life.

It's necessary to keep preventative factors in mind. For example, a patient who says their pet keeps them alive may be at increased risk of suicide if the pet gets lost or dies. Factors that increase the risk of suicide include male sex, advanced age, single marital status (or widower), lower socioeconomic status, unemployment, depression, schizophrenia, alcohol or drug abuse/dependence, and distressing life events.

Other areas that should be assessed for risk include self-harm, danger to others, vulnerability to exploitation, the likelihood of substance abuse, noncompliance with treatment, homelessness, and risk of self-neglect.

Other Investigations

The psychiatric mental health nurse should assess for a history of psychological trauma. Trauma is associated with an increased risk for psychiatric disease. The 13-item self-report trauma screening instrument is a short version of the Trauma Assessment for Adults instrument used to screen for psychological trauma. The Adverse Childhood Experiences questionnaire is used to assess for childhood trauma.

If a patient is suspected of organic cerebral pathology, other diagnostic tests, such as CT, MRI, EEG, etc., should be ordered. In young patients who have a history of drug abuse, hepatitis B and C and HIV tests should be ordered. Tests that are done when the patient presents for the first time include hepatic, renal, and thyroid function, complete blood count, and calcium and phosphate levels.

Chapter 6: Client-Centered Care

Client-centered care is also known as patient-centered care. It is a healthcare model that focuses on the patient's feelings of involvement in their treatment and care journey. Client-centered care is highly personalized for patients. The goal of client-centered care is to empower and educate patients, encourage them to make decisions about their treatment plans, create individualized plans, and improve patient outcomes.

Nurses who are educated in client-centered care use a holistic approach. They consider the well-being of the patient as a whole instead of the isolated illness. There are many definitions for client-centered care. It is important to remember that the core concept is the focus on the individual with the physical or mental health issue and how the care journey affects them. This includes all aspects of their functioning and not just treatment of the disease.

Applying client-centered care is essential in psychiatry. Psychiatric disorders affect every aspect of the patient's ability to function. Psychiatric symptoms influence a patient's interactions with family members, coworkers, and friends, their productivity in the workplace, socioeconomic status, and other important areas of life.

Principles of Client-Centered Care

The definition of client-centered care continues to evolve. Client-centered care incorporates many activities and goals that depend on the individual, their needs, and preferences. The main framework of client-centered care consists of the following principles:

Welcoming Environment

The first appointment at the psychiatrist can be intimidating for patients. The psychiatric mental health nurse practitioner should ensure the initial interaction between the patient and healthcare provider is in a safe, comfortable, welcoming environment. This is particularly emphasized for patients who are in a potential state of agitation, experiencing a panic attack, or psychosis.

Respect for the Patient's Preferences, Needs, and Values

The psychiatric mental health nurse practitioner should get to know the patient on an individual level and recognize their strengths, beliefs, perspectives, needs, and values. The patient should be treated as an active participant in their treatment plan. Information about the patient's priorities should be obtained. The patient, their family members, and caregivers should be informed of the treatment plan, prognosis, and outcomes. The psychiatric mental health nurse practitioner should aim to develop a reciprocal, mutually respectful relationship that will incorporate the patient's unique values.

Coordination and Integration of Care

The medical team that provides treatment to the patient should be organized and coordinated as much as possible. This enables a smooth and productive recovery. Transitions between different providers in different phases of treatment should not cause confusion or stress. This is especially important for patients who need various types of care. It can also limit healthcare costs, excessive medication prescriptions, unnecessary tests and screenings, and prolonged hospitalization.

Disruptive, disorganized care may cause poor outcomes. The psychiatric mental health nurse practitioner should assess the patient's need for different services that are both formal and informal. Care management and referrals should be provided as needed.

Clear Information, Education, and Support

Patients should be empowered and proactive in their treatment journey. The psychiatric mental health practitioner should educate them on the steps involved in their plan, lab results, physical findings, expected effects of medications, adverse effects of medications, etc. The patient and their families should get the information promptly. Patients should not feel as if the healthcare staff withholds information from them.

Comfort and Support

Psychiatric disorders have an impact on the emotional well-being of patients. When a patient is diagnosed with a psychiatric disorder they are often faced with stigma. The disorder might have caused them to lose their job or a significant other. Depression is a common co-morbid condition of many psychiatric disorders. The psychiatric mental health nurse practitioner should consider the patient's emotional well-being and provide care in an empathetic environment. Patients should be offered sensitivity and reassurance.

A patient may develop anxiety and depression without a support system. This can negatively affect treatment adherence. Patients may also feel lonely and isolated. The psychiatric mental health nurse practitioner should be able to address the patient's fears. These may include the impact of their disease on their life, financial costs of the disease, and anxieties related to side effects of medications.

Involvement of Family and Friends

Social support is very important for every individual. The psychiatric mental health nurse practitioner should empower the patient's family and friends and inform them of the positive impact they can have on the health of their loved one.

Sociocultural Competence

The psychiatric mental health nurse practitioner should be aware of the sociocultural background of the patient and its impact on the healthcare journey. Health literacy level might affect compliance with treatment. Economic and educational status can affect the patient's ability to participate in the treatment plan. Family situations can influence the course of illness. Culture and tradition should also be considered. The nurse should communicate at a level that the patient can understand.

Access to Care

Patients should be provided access to proper services at all times. Wait times should be minimized and service hours should be convenient. The patient should gather skills to navigate the healthcare system.

Continuity of Care and Smooth Transitions

The psychiatric mental health nurse practitioner should ensure that patients can take care of themselves after discharge. Readmissions should be reduced through attention to smooth transitions among the medical staff, care providers, and the patient's environment.

Confidentiality

Trust is necessary for a productive relationship between the healthcare provider and the patient. Making the patient feel safe and comfortable will encourage them to disclose information that they consider intimate. The patient should be informed that confidentiality will be maintained when appropriate.

Responsibility

Patients should perform as many tasks as they are able. This will increase the patient's self-esteem and develop their skills. The psychiatric mental health nurse practitioner should recognize the patient's boundaries and avoid pushing them too far.

Community Outreach

Local community outreach will make the patient feel more connected and reduce feelings of isolation. This will improve the patient's quality of life and treatment satisfaction.

Treatment of Patients with Dignity

Patients should always be treated with dignity. Medical professionals should listen to what they have to say and consider their input. The psychiatrist should avoid any shame in association with the patient's treatment. They should also avoid judgments associated with a patient's decisions. Shame may cause the patient to withhold necessary information. This may obstruct or prematurely end treatment.

Why is a Client-Centered Care Approach Needed in Psychiatry?

Current psychiatric care uses a bio-psycho-social model that is considered client-centered. Psychiatry has historically been criticized for "categorization" of individuals in terms of "mental illnesses" without proper attention to their different backgrounds, culture, religion, past trauma, and experiences. There are still barriers that must be addressed to achieve client-centered care. For example, some reports suggest that a significant number of individuals feel as if they are not completely involved in their treatment. Some studies also suggest that psychiatrists can inaccurately overestimate their work performance and collaboration.

Rights

Healthcare providers in psychiatry are often required to restrict individual freedoms of the patient to achieve the best clinical outcome. The need for involuntary hospitalization comes when a patient is a threat to themselves or others. Clinicians must achieve a balance between respecting the patient's human rights and providing the best care. The responsibility of healthcare providers is to be knowledgeable about human rights and relevant legislation. Healthcare providers should always respect people's rights and wishes, and treat them with dignity.

Implications for Practice and Service Organization

Client-centered care and personal recovery both draw attention to the patient's recovery goals. The patient's history, values, circumstances, and strengths influence the clinician's decision-making process in terms of diagnosis, support, and management plans. In client-centered care, the clinician develops the management plan in collaboration with the patient. This allows the patient to live the life they want. The implication of using this approach is that sometimes the practitioner might have to adapt treatments to fit the patient's individual preferences and circumstances, even if it means deviating from strict adherence to current and evidence-based guidelines.

Implications for Healthcare Providers

The client-centered care approach aims to improve the lives of healthcare providers. Healthcare providers working in psychiatry are at risk of burn-out. This influences the clinician's well-being and quality of life as well as the clinical outcomes. For doctors and nurses to be able to treat people with compassion, respect, and dignity, they should work in well-organized services that can recognize their needs. The client-centered care approach improves work satisfaction and reduces burn-out levels. The well-being of healthcare providers is a major factor in the delivery of optimal care.

Values and Evidence

The practice of evidence-based medicine incorporates clinical guidelines and protocols. However, in a client-centered care approach, the clinical decision process should not be based on inflexible use of guidelines and protocols. There should be collaboration between healthcare providers and patients to ensure that care is tailored to the individual's specific situation and needs. Client-centered care is delivered when both evidence-based practice and values-based practice are respected. The core values include dignity, empathy, fairness, humility, honesty, trust, and respect.

Training

The current curriculum for trainees in psychiatry does not properly include client-centered care and its capabilities. For future professionals to incorporate client-centered care in their treatment, the curriculum should include elements such as:

- Language that reflects client-centered care.
- Relational competencies that include self-directed support, co-production, shared decision-making, support-planning, etc.
- Competencies that are related to client-centered care such as social inclusion, human rights, community engagement, and other legislation.

Summative and formative assessments should be done to motivate trainees to learn.

Example of Client-Centered Care

Case Vignette

Maria is a 55-year-old kindergarten teacher. In the past month, she has suffered from decreased mood. She describes her problems as lack of focus, inability to fall asleep, lack of interest in activities that used to bring her pleasure, feelings of worthlessness and guilt, and lack of appetite. She reports that she has lost five pounds in the past month. She complains that she finds it hard to finish tasks at work and feels like she has failed the children in her care.

Maria's psychiatrist listens to her complaints, simultaneously assesses her physical appearance, and conducts a mental status examination. She notices her psychomotor activity, speech, and affect. She continues to ask questions to gain more clarity about her condition. The psychiatrist checks the criteria of major depressive disorder to properly diagnose Maria. She also asks Maria questions about her life and her nature as a person. She asks her how her family members and friends have reacted to her condition, whether she has a strong social support system, and if any environmental stressors in her life might make her condition worse.

Maria's psychiatrist shows interest in getting to know her patients better. She learns about the role the psychiatric disorder has in Maria's life. She expresses empathy and encourages Maria to collaborate with her to develop a treatment plan. She informs Maria of medications that will be used to treat her condition and potential adverse effects. Maria and her psychiatrist stay in touch during treatment. At every follow-up visit, the psychiatrist informs Maria of progress and expectations for the future.

The psychiatrist respects the principles of client-centered care through interest in her patient as a whole and not just an isolated illness. She is interested in the patient's life and treats Maria with respect, compassion, and dignity. With a client-centered care approach, the psychiatrist can build a mutually collaborative relationship with her patient. This will improve the patient's outcomes as well as the doctor's job satisfaction and success.

Chapter 7: Educational Concepts

The psychiatric mental health nurse practitioner should provide patients with clear instructions on how to manage their mental and overall health after discharge from treatment. Patients should be educated on how to self-monitor symptoms as well as maintain healthy habits, lifestyle changes, and other healing modalities that will improve their outcome. Patient education takes skill, compassion, patience, and commitment. Barriers that can influence patient education include hectic shifts and lack of available resources. Nurses can increase patient education with motivation for positive change. Nurses should be aware of the basic principles of learning to understand how a person can be educated in the most effective way.

Basic Principles of Learning

The process of learning can be impacted by factors such as the meaningfulness of the material, retention, transfer of learning, and individual factors. Primary individual factors include the age of the individual, intelligence, previous learning, anxiety, and motivation.

Intelligence has many theories and definitions. It can be defined as the capacity of the individual to learn new information and use that information. A combination of inherent and acquired capabilities influences an individual's intelligence level.

Age and maturation are significant factors that affect learning. For an individual to learn, they must be ready to do so. Learning has a hierarchical component. This means that new knowledge is built upon previous knowledge and new and old knowledge is connected. This hierarchical nature has an especially big influence on children as their learning is largely dependent on age and maturation.

Education level is another factor that influences learning. The amount of a person's accumulated knowledge significantly contributes to the ease and speed of learning new material. This is especially accentuated if the new material is related to something previously learned.

Psychologists have attempted to define factors that influence a person's motivation to learn. According to Murray, the need for achievement is one of the psychological needs that drive the motivation to learn. According to Maslow, the individual has basic psychological needs (such as water, sleep, food, safety, and oxygen). As these needs are fulfilled, the individual progresses to higher-level needs, including those for self-actualization. Other motivational influences include goals, interests, reinforcements, incentives, and drive determinants.

The level of anxiety an individual experiences is another factor that impacts the process of learning. Individuals may feel afraid of failure, lack self-confidence, or have a low degree of self-efficacy. All these factors impact a person's ability to learn. Anxiety can elicit various responses. For example, someone who fears failure may feel hopeless. This can result in unwillingness to learn new content. Some people who are afraid of failure may overcompensate with greater effort so they do not fail. Past failures and successes are projected onto present situations. This influences how people respond and learn.

Methods

Presentation of material is an important factor in the learning process. Though there are variations in people's abilities and motivations to learn, certain methods can maximize the effectiveness and efficiency of learning for most people. These methods have an impact on recall, transfer, and retention. The most important methods include active participation, distribution of practice, whole versus part, and knowledge of results.

Active participation increases an individual's ability to learn cognitive and psychomotor tasks. By taking an active role in the learning process, people can understand better, develop their skills, and increase their ability for retention. Examples of active participation include paying attention, pattern recognition, searching for relationships in the material, comments, questions, thought regarding the presented content, and practicing skills.

To achieve optimal learning of a skill, practice time must be properly distributed for sufficient length. It should also be arranged in a way that enables continuity between response and reinforcement. This can be achieved through frequent practice sessions, sequencing tasks, and emphasis on accuracy over speed.

People learn better when they have an image of the whole before its discrete parts. A review of the entire task facilitates knowledge of how each part fits and its use. Tasks should be divided into smaller, manageable units. This will make it easier for learners to focus and not feel overwhelmed.

The provision of results and constructive feedback facilitates the learning process. People feel encouraged to do better when they receive input about their performance. Input enables people to acknowledge their strengths and identify and correct potential errors.

Meaningfulness of Material

Motivation for learning is increased when the material has meaning for the learners. Meaningfulness and associations with the material increase the motivation for participation. Individuals can make associations with material they have previously learned, with their needs or drives, or with emotional content. Associations can be made with the material through its organization into conceptual categories.

Transfer of Learning

The transfer of learning is divided into horizontal and vertical transfer. Vertical transfer occurs when the individual uses old concepts to understand or learn concepts with an increased complexity. Horizontal transfer occurs when a new task is performed at the same level of complexity as an old task. The formal discipline theory of transfer is built upon the idea of universal study of mathematics, logic, Greek, and Latin. These disciplines train the mind with their complexity. People train the mind with practice of difficult subjects just as exercise trains the body. The theory of identical elements states that transfer occurs from one learning to another when the two materials have common elements. If the materials are very different, then the amount of transfer decreases.

Retention

For material to have any use for the learner, they must be able to learn and retain it. Many factors influence whether someone will forget what they have learned. People tend to easily forget material that has no meaning for them. The trace decay theory of forgetting states that people retain and strengthen memories that they use. Memories that are not being used gradually fade away. The interference theory states that proactive inhibition causes forgetting when previous learning interferes with the learning of new material. Retroactive inhibition happens when new material interferes with the retrieval of previous material.

The rate of forgetting is influenced by the degree to which the person has learned the material, how relevant the material is to the needs of the person, the actions connected to the material after the learning, and the physical and psychological state of the person during learning and recall. Retention is increased when the material is thoroughly learned, the material has meaning for the learner, the learner uses the material after learning it, and there are no intervening situations that are traumatic enough to interfere.

The curve of forgetting is determined by how much of the material is forgotten after the learning process and how the material is remembered over time.

Goals

The clinician should develop goals for the individual or psychoeducational group. An educational component is especially important. The goals should be direct, clear, and specific. To develop goals, it's best to consider the needs, readiness, and motivations of the learners. Sometimes this can be hard to achieve if the clinician does not have much information about the individuals or participants before the first meeting. However, some general concepts can be helpful for this task. The clinician should develop and review these goals with the patient and make sure they agree. They should inquire of the patient whether they think the goals are appropriate, if they have any changes to suggest, and if they agree to work towards them.

Assessment of Learning Needs

Assessment of the patient's learning needs is the first process in patient education. This can determine what they already know, what they want to learn, what they need to learn, what they are capable of learning, and effective teaching methods. The clinician should find out more about the patient as an individual. This can be achieved with questions about their typical day, family, work, etc. The patient's needs can be assessed with questions about their main concerns and goals, what they need to achieve their goals, their specific problems, what they are the most interested in, etc.

Assessment of Learning Style

Assessment of the patient's learning style will help match teaching strategies so learning is more effective. Helpful information may include the patient's preferred time for learning, if they prefer to read or watch a video, or if they want the material to be explained to them before they interact with it. It's also important to know whether they have any problems that would prevent them from learning new material.

Any missing information can be obtained from the patient's family. Conversations with family members can help you understand the patient's home situation and assess whether the family is supportive of the patient's wish to change their behavior. Checklists and questionnaires can be used to gather more information about the patient's learning style. Collaboration with the healthcare team can provide valuable information about what type of teaching strategies to use.

Development of Learning Objectives

Learning objectives are short-term, attainable, and measurable. Goal achievement can be made easier if goals are broken down into learning objectives. An example of a learning objective is, "After this meeting, the patient will be able to identify the symptoms of depression." This is a step towards a larger goal. Development of learning objectives should use measurable terms such as explain, list, or demonstrate.

Readiness to Learn

Readiness to learn refers to the patient's willingness to gather knowledge and implement behavioral changes. Patients usually go through several stages to adopt a new behavior:

1. During the pre-contemplative stage the patient is not aware that they have a problem and may not be ready to act.
2. In the contemplative stage the patient starts to consider change but is still not ready to take action.
3. In the action stage the patient starts to practice a behavior change and learn how to maintain it.
4. During the maintenance stage the patient reinforces the learned behavior and it becomes a part of their everyday life.

The clinician's interventions are most effective if they match the patient's readiness to learn. For example, if the patient is not aware that they have a problem then psychoeducation should become a goal to increase the patient's awareness. Patients who have a willingness and readiness to learn will be more receptive to the clinician's teaching efforts. Readiness to learn is influenced by physical comfort, such as the presence of pain. Psychological comfort is also an influence as it pertains to anxiety, fear, and calmness. Teaching material should be matched to the patient's stage of readiness. This can be assessed with direct questions about what the patient thinks regarding their healthcare problem and what actions they would like to take.

Chapter 8: Cultural Competence

Culture can be defined as a way of living in a specific society that consists of shared patterns of belief, knowledge, and feelings that influence people's behavior. These patterns are passed down through generations. Ethnicity refers to a common identity among people because of a shared heritage. Culture and ethnicity affect human behavior.

In the United States, there is a large number of immigrants, descendants of immigrants, and foreign-born residents. This number increases every year. To be able to work with the diverse US population and understand the impact of cultural influences, nurses must obtain knowledge of cultural concepts and ethnicity. However, nurses should be careful not to assume that all people from the same cultural or ethnic groups exhibit the same behavior. This is called stereotyping. There are many variations and subcultures that exist within a culture. These variations may be due to status, residence, religion, education, ethnic background, etc. Every patient's uniqueness must be appreciated. Culturally competent care is a way to minimize misunderstandings that may arise between healthcare providers and patients due to cultural diversity. Nurses who practice with cultural competence understand and acknowledge cultural differences. They also respond to every patient's different customs, languages, and beliefs.

Cultural Competence in Different Populations

Native Americans

There are 574 American Indian tribes and Alaska Native groups currently recognized by the federal government. Native Americans may appear as reserved and silent people who do not express much emotion. Their culture considers that private thoughts should be kept to oneself. Some Native Americans consider the classic handshake to be too aggressive. Eye contact may also be considered rude.

In their living space, nuclear and extended families often live together. The family and the tribe are the main social organizations. Traditions are valued and passed down from elders to children. Religion and health are combined. The healer is called the shaman. The shaman uses many methods in their healing practices such as a crystal to diagnose disease, songs, healing ceremonies, and plants, roots, and herbs with healing properties. The Native American healers collaborate with the US Indian Health Service. Native American healers communicate with physicians regarding the care of some patients.

Native Americans are at higher risk of illness and premature death from diabetes, tuberculosis, heart disease, suicide, pneumonia, influenza, homicide, automobile accidents, and substance abuse. They have higher rates of depression and other problems such as spouse and child abuse. Alcoholism is a significant issue.

African Americans

Some African Americans have a different dialect than standard English. They often have large social support systems which include brothers, sisters, uncles, aunts, cousins, neighbors, friends, etc. African Americans value religious life and most practice some form of Protestantism. There are still patterns of discrimination in the US that date back to slavery. Black neighborhoods, churches, and schools are evidence of historical segregation and other socioeconomic issues.

Some African Americans who have encountered racism and discrimination may have difficulties with planning future goals due to a sense of hopelessness. They may struggle with unemployment and low-paying jobs. They may have little hope or expectation for improvement of their economic situation.

Asian/Pacific Islander Americans

Asian Americans consist of people from areas such as Japan, China, Thailand, Cambodia, Korea, India, Laos, the Pacific Islands, and the Philippines. People from these cultures have various attitudes, values, religious practices, and languages. They may share similar beliefs regarding interaction between people. For example, raising one's voice as a sign of lost control or touch during conversation may be unacceptable. Eye contact may be seen as a lack of respect.

Loyalty to the family is considered important. Children are often taught to respect their elders. There may be associated shame for individuals who suffer from mental illness. Many individuals may present with somatic complaints which may be more acceptable than expression of true emotions.

Latino Americans

Latino Americans comprise the largest ethnic minority group in the United States. They trace their ancestry back to Central and South American countries such as Puerto Rico, Cuba, and Mexico. Spanish is a common language with several dialects. Latinos may use a lot of touch in their communication. Their primary social organization is the family. The family typically includes both members from the nuclear family and extended family members.

Religion may have a strong influence on their lives which may increase during times of crisis. Folk beliefs associated with health are influenced by Roman Catholicism, Spanish, and Indian beliefs. Common treatments among folk healers may include diet, indigenous herbs, prayers, massage, rest, supernatural rituals, and practical advice.

Research suggests that among Latino Americans there is less mental illness compared to the general population. This may be due to the strong cohesion of family and social support.

Arab Americans

The ancestry of Arab Americans can be traced back to various countries in the Arab world, including the Arabian Peninsula, North Africa, and the Levant. Their official language is Arabic and English is a common second language. Communication and language can be barriers in healthcare settings for patients from Arabic countries.

The main social organization is the family. The modesty of women is valued. Many Muslim women practice the hijab which covers the whole body except the face and hands.

Islam is the religion of many Arabic people. Some Muslim people believe in the combination of conventional medicine with spiritual medicine. Part of healing is done through daily prayers and words from the Qur'an.

There may be stigma around mental illness in the Arabic community. Many people who suffer from mental distress may present with vague somatic complaints.

LGBTQ+ Patients

The LGBTQ+ community (lesbian, gay, bisexual, transgender, queer/questioning) includes members from all races, ethnicities, socioeconomic status, and religious backgrounds. To provide culturally competent care for LGBTQ+ individuals, healthcare providers should avoid discrimination, stigmatization, and unconscious biases. They should aim for equality of care.

LGBTQ+ individuals may be faced with various psychosocial stressors and challenges throughout their lives. Healthcare educators should be aware of important issues as well as the proper usage of terms as determined by the LGBTQ+ community. They should never use derogatory words at any time.

Some challenges that healthcare providers may have with care of LGBTQ+ patients include difficulties in open discussion of sexual health-related problems. Care should be taken to use gender-neutral terms and supportive language. Providers can create a practice that welcomes patients of the LGBTQ+ community through education of their staff and an open-minded and nonjudgmental environment.

LGBTQ+ patients have a higher risk of mental health issues and trauma due to violence compared to their heterosexual peers. They may have higher rates of substance abuse and depression which may be due to the stress of discrimination. Adolescents who are a part of a sexual and gender minority have a higher suicide rate. Social support and community connectedness can reduce this risk. Affirmative psychotherapy can reduce the negative impact of homophobia and transphobia and strengthen a positive view of LGBTQ relationships and identities.

Remember that members of the LGBTQ+ community may want to keep their gender or sexual orientation private. Confidentiality must be guaranteed. The HIPAA Privacy Rule states that the provider must respect the patient's wishes on matters related to privacy.

Chapter 9: Communication Barrier Management

The previous chapter addressed cultural competence in mental health nursing. The patient's culture has an impact on the successful communication between the patient and healthcare provider. Awareness of communication barriers can help nurses better navigate the therapeutic process with patients from all backgrounds. This chapter will address communication barriers and ways to successfully manage them.

Time Constraints

The lack of time can be a significant barrier to communication. Rushed meetings are less effective. However, nurses may be pressured with time constraints due to heavy demand. Quality communication does not always have to be time-consuming. Simple "small talk" or a smile may help build rapport with patients. It's best to take time to get to know patients on a more personal level to be better prepared for potentially difficult conversations that may arise.

In pressured clinics or wards there may be interruptions or delays in conversations between healthcare providers and patients. This is usually due to the needs of other patients. This may frustrate some patients and make them feel neglected. When interruptions happen, it is best to explain to patients that you must leave and arrange a time for your return.

Environmental Factors

Sometimes healthcare providers get used to their environment and may not notice environmental factors that can cause communication difficulties. Busy clinics with a lot of background noise can impair patients' hearing. Some patients may pretend that they can hear by nodding. When you notice that a patient is not hearing well, you should make an effort to reduce the background noise. You can try to find a quiet corner or go to a quieter room. Notice if the patient is wearing any hearing aids. If so, check for proper function.

Patients with dementia often have cognitive impairments and difficulties with concentration. Noise and distractions can significantly impact communication with these patients. The communication of important information with these patients should be planned. Important conversations should take place in the best time and place possible.

Patients will not disclose sensitive information if they feel like other people can hear them. Avoid discussion of sensitive information within other people's earshot. Written forms may be used in certain cases. Some patients who do not understand the language may need a professional interpreter to translate the form for them.

Distress and Fatigue

Patients who experience distress, pain, or fatigue may have difficulties with concentration. This can affect the information-gathering process. If it is important to obtain information in a moment when a patient is in distress, it's helpful to acknowledge their discomfort and explain the need for communication. Use a statement such as, "I know you are not feeling very well right now, but we need to talk."

Some patients are not fully alert. This can make communication especially difficult. You should decide if it is necessary to have the conversation right away or if some parts of the message can be delivered now and other parts later. If patients are unable to give their full attention, break down information into smaller parts so it is easier to digest. Ask patients if they need you to repeat the information. Acknowledgement of the patient's distress can build rapport and make the patient more communicative. If the information is very important, you can have the patient repeat the information back to you.

Embarrassment and Anxiety

Patients may feel embarrassed to talk about sensitive information such as difficult family situations, addiction, sexual dysfunction, etc. Embarrassment can reduce the effectiveness of communication. However, there are ways to minimize potential embarrassment.

Notice any signs of embarrassment in your patient such as blushing, laughter, fidgeting, joking, or other behaviors that aim to mask embarrassment. Use positive and open body language when talking to patients. This will make them feel more comfortable.

You should avoid judgmental statements since they may increase embarrassment. Ask questions in a neutral and open way for information. This will elicit more honest answers and information.

Patients may feel reluctant to ask for clarification or more information if they see it as a waste of time. Let them know that their health is your priority and that there are no stupid questions. You can encourage them to ask questions with, "I know you have questions. Is there anything that you would like me to answer for you?"

Jargon

Technical jargon and clinical acronyms are helpful in communication between healthcare providers. However, you should avoid the use of technical jargon in front of patients. This requires conscious effort since it is easy to slip jargon into a conversation without realization. When patients hear technical terms, they may be reluctant to admit that they do not understand what has been said.

Avoid using ambiguous terms. Some words may have different meanings for the patient. The vocabulary should be appropriate for the specific audience. Do not use childish expressions with elderly patients. If the patient is not fluent in English, avoid complex sentences and slang. Try to speak more slowly. Avoid discussion of statistics since this may confuse some patients.

Values, Beliefs, Assumptions

Everyone has different assumptions, values, cultural beliefs, biases, and prejudices. Some patients may find it hard to believe that a man can be a nurse or that a doctor can be female. Notice assumptions that can cause misinterpretations. Some assumptions may cause a patient to ignore you. You can solve these situations with an introduction of yourself and your role, "Hello, I am your mental health nurse practitioner and I will be examining you today."

Nurses can also be affected by their assumptions, values, and beliefs. This can impact communication with patients. Patients may get offended by incorrect assumptions.

Information Overload

People can become confused when bombarded with a lot of information. This is especially true for patients who struggle with anxiety, distress, or pain. When you need to provide a patient with a lot of information, notice how they are feeling. You can point out that some information is important for them to hear.

When you need to have a complex conversation with a lot of new information, you can ask the patient to bring a family member or a friend so they can both hear it. Be mindful that some patients do not want other people to know about their mental health issues.

You can encourage patients to take notes if they wish. If the patient is comfortable, you can record the conversation so they can hear it again at a later time. You can also provide patients with written information to supplement what has been said. Arrange another meeting if there is a need to repeat information or share additional details.

Language and Culture

Cultural norms and customs influence the way we think and express ourselves. Expression of communication is done through language (speaking and writing), paralanguage (speed of speech, intonation, voice quality, rhythm), and gestures (facial expression, body posture, eye movements, physical appearance, touch). When there is a language barrier between a healthcare provider and the patient, an interpreter might be necessary. Interpretation involves translation, but it also requires knowledge of and sensitivity to cultural nuances.

Certain tips can make an interpreter more effective. Speak directly to the patient instead of through the interpreter. Maintain eye contact with the patient to keep them involved. When the patient and interpreter speak, do not interrupt them. Their interactions may require more time due to dialect differences or a need for more extensive clarifications. The interpreter might need to prepare the patient before the next question.

Instruct the interpreter to translate with the same words as the patient so you can understand their thoughts and feelings. Avoid using technical jargon which may be difficult for both patient and interpreter to understand. Avoid long conversations with the interpreter in front of the patient. This can make the patient feel left out and ignored.

Intimate and emotional topics may need to be discussed. This may be difficult for both the patient and the interpreter. Ask the patient for permission to discuss these topics. Lead up to them slowly. You should prepare the interpreter for the emotional nature of these interviews.

If possible, allow the patient and interpreter to meet before the interview to build rapport. This can be positive for the interview process. If possible, use the same interpreter for subsequent interviews with the same patient.

It's best to use an interpreter who is similar in age to the patient. Make a list of questions that you plan to ask beforehand. Inform the interpreter what you plan to ask before the meeting with the patient. During the interview, address the questions to the patient and not the interpreter.

Culture-Based Communication

Communication issues may arise due to cultural differences. Mental health nurses work with patients from multicultural backgrounds. They should be aware of the influence of culture on communication. Patients from different backgrounds can behave and communicate in various ways with different rules for communication. For example, eye contact is considered disrespectful in some cultural groups.

Different cultural groups may have different terms for mental health issues. Factors that motivate communication such as rules and rituals also vary between different cultural groups. Beliefs influence communication and may be part of discussions.

Collectivism and individualism are different across cultures. Patients from collectivist cultures may believe their successes are due to individual strengths and their failures are due to external circumstances.

The patient's culture may influence the extent of their self-disclosure. Some cultures are more private with intimate information. Periods of silence can be interpreted differently. For example, some cultures consider silence as passive aggression. Non-verbal communication such as handshakes or physical contact varies between cultures as well.

The mental health nurse should be aware of their prejudices and biases. They should explore how culture influences the behaviors, thoughts, and feelings of patients.

Chapter 10: Treatment Planning

Elements of Treatment Planning

Treatment planning is a structured process. It requires an organized effort to create a program to outline what should happen when patients are provided with the most effective treatment. The treatment plan should be tailored to the various needs of individual patients. There are many different approaches to the development of a treatment plan. Most treatment plans share common elements which include identification and background information, a list of problems, goals, and objectives, intervention strategies and tactics, and flexibility.

Identification and Background Information

The treatment plan starts with basic information about the patient (e.g., name, age, employment status, and marital status), reasons for treatment, and previous medical and psychiatric history. Information regarding current medical and psychiatric health issues, diagnoses, and treatments should also be included.

Referral Source and Reason for Referral

It is important to identify the individual or organization that referred the patient for treatment and the reason for the referral. Patients often recognize that they have a problem and manage to seek out resources or contact a health provider who will help them cope. These patients are self-referred. In some cases, someone else who is aware of the patient's problem makes the referral. Examples of these cases include friends of the patient, physicians, crisis intervention workers, courts, school systems, parents, and others who can identify that the patient has a problem.

Presentation of the Problem

The treatment plan includes the current problem that requires treatment. The main complaint should be written in the patient's own words. The way in which the patient describes the problem can provide clearer information about it, its intensity, and the effect it has on the patient's life as compared to the clinician's description. See the following example of the patient's description. "I came here because life has been feeling extra hard lately. I cannot get out of bed and I keep having nightmares that I'm going to lose my job. It just does not seem worth it to keep on living anymore." Compare this to the doctor's description. "The patient suffers from anxiety and depression." Obviously, the patient's description conveys more information.

It is important to remember that the written plan serves to communicate important information to other healthcare providers. Therefore, if the patient's statement is not clear enough the clinician can provide additional clarification.

Problem List

The clinician can identify various problems with thorough assessment of the patient. The patient and clinician should work together to identify and prioritize the most significant problems to work on during treatment. The problems should be defined in a way that presents how they manifest themselves in the patient and their life. The problems included in this section should have a significant impact on the patient's daily life and ability to function in terms of work, school, social life, and family. The problems should be addressable with a health intervention.

The problems should be written in clear and non-ambiguous language. For example, "school problems" is not descriptive enough as it may have different meanings for different patients. Better descriptions include "undisciplined behavior during class," "aggressive behavior towards peers," or "academic underachievement." Clear and extensive descriptions enable the clinician to pinpoint the problem to be the focus of the intervention.

Prioritization of Problems

The problem list can vary in length among patients. All of the problems should be well understood and communicated in clear language. The problems listed are what impair the patient's ability to function in an important area of life and are responsive to a psychological, psychiatric, or other health intervention. After confirmation, the clinician should prioritize the problems as a guide to which the treatment should address first.

In prioritization of problems, consider the degree and extent to which they impact the patient's life. However, you should not lose sight of the broader picture as there may be one reason for the patient's problems. Management of the cause can alleviate the other interconnected problems.

There are a few questions that will help you prioritize the problem list. These include:

- Is there a threat to the patient or others?
- Is there a problem that will jeopardize the therapy?
- Is there a problem that if unresolved will block solutions to other problems?
- Which problem has the most impact on the patient's life?
- Which problem's solution will resolve many of the other problems?
- Is there a problem that is easily solvable?
- Which problem is the patient most committed to solving?
- Is there a lower-priority problem that should be addressed later?

The first question is a top priority. Any situations that pose a danger to the patient or others must be addressed first. These include suicidality, homicidality, domestic violence, substance abuse or dependence, and neglect of children or other people the patient is responsible for.

Limit the Length of the Problem List

Clinicians often take care of patients who have many problems. Solutions to all the problems might be impossible due to various reasons. These include limitations of the healthcare plan benefits, reluctance of the patient to be engaged in treatment for an extended time, and other factors. Clinician factors that can affect the length of treatment include limited practice hours, potential practice closure, and others. In these situations, the clinician should limit the problem list to those that are highly prioritized and can be effectively treated under the circumstances.

Diagnosis

Assignment of the correct diagnosis is necessary for many reasons. A diagnosis is required for reimbursement from third-party payers. The treatments described in the literature are linked to diagnoses. A correct diagnosis will help the clinician choose the most appropriate treatment. A diagnosis can also predict the course and prognosis of the condition.

Diagnoses that are based on accepted diagnostic classification systems make communication easier between healthcare providers and other parties. The diagnostic classification system is chosen by the payer of the treatment. The most-used system is the DSM-5. In some cases, the ICD-10 is required. However, the DSM-5 is the most familiar among healthcare providers. It is also taught in residencies, internships, and graduate school courses.

Goals and Objectives

Objectives are a series of steps that need to be completed in order to achieve a desired goal. Objectives need to be objective, measurable, and short-term. Goals are long-term and do not have to be measurable. To develop and implement goals and objectives, clinicians can use the SMART (Specific, Measurable, Achievable, Realistic, and Time-limited) goals approach.

Specific

Specific goals can be measured. For example, if a person who suffers from social anxiety says that their goal is to “feel better,” that is a nonspecific goal that would be difficult to measure. If their goal is to have at least one conversation with a stranger per day, that goal is specific. It can be a challenge to monitor a patient’s progress if goals are nonspecific.

Measurable

Objectives should be measurable. Goals should be put in measurable terms. Measurable means specific, quantifiable, and easy to understand. Measurability allows you to track and monitor the patient’s progress. This informs you whether the chosen treatment is effective and helps you decide if any adjustments to the treatment are necessary. With this information, patients can see how much they have progressed since they began treatment. It can also motivate them to continue to actively participate.

Achievable

If the patient can accomplish the goal with the given circumstances and resources, that goal is achievable. If the goal is achievable, you should determine whether the patient can reach it within a reasonable timeline.

Clinicians may be faced with patients who want to accomplish unachievable goals. An example of an unachievable goal is a patient diagnosed with chronic schizophrenia who has a goal to work at a high-stress job in a stock brokerage firm without adequate support and treatment. To end alcohol abuse is an achievable goal but is unlikely to be reached in one week.

Unachievable goals should be avoided regardless of any pressure that third parties might put on the clinician. That can increase the likelihood of failure and possible early termination of treatment.

Realistic

Once you have determined that the patient can achieve a certain goal or objective in a specified amount of time, the next factor is whether that goal, objective, or timeline is realistic. The patient must have enough motivation to put in the required work. They should have family members and significant others to provide enough support. The patient's insurance company should pay for the treatment. The reality of the situation must always be considered. An unrealistic goal results in negative outcomes.

Time-limited

Having a timeline for completion of the goal shows that the clinician believes the patient can achieve it in a timely fashion. This can increase the patient's self-esteem, motivation, and will to achieve the set goals and objectives.

Users of the Treatment Plan

The Treating Clinician

The clinician is the main audience for the treatment plan. It will guide the progress of treatment and is a tool that enables the clinician to facilitate the therapeutic intervention. The clinician will use the treatment plan more than anyone else. In most cases, the clinician who develops the treatment plan is the one who is responsible for the patient. In other cases, there should be clear and consistent communication between the healthcare providers to avoid any misunderstandings.

The Patient

The patient should agree to the problems that have been identified, the treatment goals and objectives, and therapeutic interventions. The treatment plan is a source of reassurance for the patient. The treatment plan can hold both patient and clinician accountable for the roles they have agreed to before treatment begins.

Insurers

Insurers may require the treatment plan to ensure the quality of care or as a formality. The treatment plan conveys information that acknowledges the health plan member will receive appropriate and adequate care. It also provides evidence that the treatment is medically necessary.

Other Third-Party Stakeholders

Other parties may have a stake in the patient's treatment. This depends on their current life circumstances. The interested party may request the submission of a treatment plan. The written plan may differ from the "standard" treatment plan as the clinician may need to modify the terminology and language to make it understandable for the third party. The third party may want to know how much recovery is expected from the therapeutic intervention.

Issues that third parties are interested in are related to the patient's potential to cause harm to others and their ability to benefit from treatment. These issues should be properly addressed in the treatment plan. Examples of third parties that may be interested in the treatment plan include courts, state vocational rehabilitation agencies, other organizations or agencies that oversee law enforcement officers, students who are evaluated for special education services, the military, the clergy, etc.

Chapter 11: Treatment Modalities

Trauma-Informed Care

Trauma-informed care is a mental healthcare approach that takes into account the impact of psychological trauma on patients and staff. It aims to provide care in a way that will not cause re-traumatization. Trauma-informed care should be applied regardless of a known history of trauma.

Individuals who have experienced trauma and stress can negatively engage with healthcare services. There is a chance of re-traumatization when a trauma survivor interacts with the healthcare system. Trauma-informed care enables healthcare providers to understand the impact of trauma on their patients. They can adapt to the needs of trauma survivors in order to improve clinical outcomes.

Trauma-informed care is based on physical and emotional safety, trustworthiness and transparency, use of peer support, cultural, historical, and gender responsiveness, and empowerment, voice, and choice. Nurses who implement trauma-informed care should be aware, responsive, and sensitive. This section presents a few practical tips to implement trauma-informed care in your nursing practice.

Practical Tips to Implement Trauma-Informed Care

Introduce Yourself and Your Role in Every Interaction
Patients have a lot of interactions with medical staff during their care. They might forget your role which may cause confusion. Therefore, it is productive to remind them of your role in their care.

Use Open and Non-Threatening Body Positions
Patients with a history of trauma might be reminded of past experiences when they interact with a provider with a threatening body posture. This may trigger feelings of powerlessness. Providers should be aware of their body language and use a non-threatening body position to help patients stay in a regulated state. Keep your body at the same level as the patient in order to reduce any chance of perceived power difference. The patient and the provider should both have access to the door to avoid feeling trapped.

Provide Anticipatory Guidance
Inform the patient what they can expect. For example, inform them that they will have several laboratory tests, visits from the resident doctors, etc. Patients with trauma are not comfortable with surprises due to unpredictability of past trauma. With information about the healthcare plan, they will feel more in control and regulated.

Ask Before Touch
Physical touch can be associated with unpleasant traumatic memories. This can activate the fight, flight, freeze response in trauma survivors. The nurse should ask for

permission before touching patients in all circumstances. This includes performance of a task multiple times in a day (e.g., when measuring a patient's blood pressure).

Protect Patient Privacy

Patients have the right to privacy. They should be able to choose the people who will be physically present during their care. If there are people in the room that the patient does not feel comfortable with (e.g., other members of the staff), the nurse should ask them to leave. The responsibility to ask others to leave should not be put on the patient as they may not feel empowered to do so.

Use Plain Language and Teach Back

It is best to use clear and simple language to communicate with patients. Avoid medical jargon. Patients who are triggered may have difficulty with the information-processing parts of the brain. This might make it difficult for them to understand and learn new information. Use of plain language empowers them and enables them to understand their care.

Recovery Model

The recovery model is a mental health approach to recovery. It highlights the belief that people can recover from mental illness through emphasis of the main components of the recovery process. These include hope, spirituality, empowerment, connection, purpose, and self-identity.

Hope is the driving force of recovery. When patients have hope they believe that change is possible. They are able to accept the problem and commit to work on changes. Hope enables people to focus on their strengths, believe in themselves, look forward and cultivate optimism, and redefine their priorities.

Spirituality can bring hope and meaning to a person's life after they have survived a stressful event. For many people, diagnosis of a severe mental illness can be a source of anxiety and stress.

Many patients with psychiatric disorders may feel helpless and dependent on mental health services. Empowerment can make them feel as if they have more control. Empowerment involves autonomy, courage, personal responsibility, and the same rights as other people without a mental illness. Patients' self-sufficiency can be empowered with appropriate income and housing, adequate access to healthcare, and freedom from violence. An empowered patient develops confidence to make independent decisions and care for themselves in their mental healthcare journey.

Close friends, families, and relationships with people in the community that believe in the individual's power to recover can be very empowering. Patients should not be isolated. Effort should be made to enable the patient to maintain close, supportive relationships.

Humans have a basic need for purpose and meaning. Patients who suffer from a psychiatric illness may struggle with a sense of purpose. They may have to give up previous goals and plans. Patients can reassess their values and find new meaning in alternative goals. This process can be made easier if patients involve themselves in work, move toward other meaningful roles, and take the time for recreational activities.

Mental illness can damage one's sense of self. Re-development of a lost sense of self is a very important part of the journey to recovery. The self should be separated from the illness. With acceptance and grief for what was lost, the patient can re-establish their identity and develop self-respect.

Cognitive Behavioral Therapy (CBT)

Cognitive behavioral therapy is based on the cognitive model. This states that people's perceptions and reactions to situations are shaped by cognitive structures. These structures are also called schemas. They are the beliefs people have about themselves, the world around them, and the future. This is called the cognitive triad.

Cognitive schemas are developed by the person's life experiences and are dependent upon their constitution. According to the cognitive model, emotional distress and negative experiences can cause the development of negative cognitive patterns. Their development is associated with many psychiatric disorders such as depression, anxiety disorder, panic disorder, personality disorders, obsessive-compulsive disorders, and somatoform disorders. The correction of negative, maladaptive cognitive structures can improve the patient's symptoms and condition.

The cognitive theory of depression states that people with depression have a negative view of self, the future, and a negative interpretation of their experiences. For example, if a student studies for a test and then fails, their perceptions may be influenced by negative cognitive structures. They may conclude, "I failed the test because I am not smart enough for this college" (negative view of self). "It's pointless to even try because these exams are so difficult. I should just give up" (negative view of the future). "I will never succeed at anything. I will fail all my exams" (negative view of experiences).

Cognitive Techniques

The cognitive approach of CBT includes identification of maladaptive assumptions, test of the validity of maladaptive assumptions, elicitation of automatic thoughts, and test of automatic thoughts.

Elicitation of automatic thoughts is done through identification of automatic cognitive distortions that occur in between the external event and the person's reaction to an event. An example of a cognitive distortion is all-or-nothing thinking.

The therapist should teach the patient how to test and carefully examine exaggerated automatic thoughts and generate alternative explanations for events. For example, the student should consider that maybe he failed the exam because he was distracted by other work and next time he can try to focus better.

Maladaptive assumptions can guide the patient's life and cause development of a psychiatric disorder such as depression. An example of a maladaptive assumption is that one must be the best at everything to deserve love.

The validity of maladaptive assumptions is tested in a similar way as automatic thoughts. Sometimes the therapist can ask the patient to defend the maladaptive assumption. For example, the patient might say that they must always be the best at everything they do and the therapist can ask why that is so important to them.

Behavioral Techniques

Behavioral techniques are used to change and test maladaptive cognitions. They help patients challenge the inaccuracy of their maladaptive cognitive structures. They also help to develop new, more adaptive ways to deal with issues. Behavioral techniques include homework assignments such as a journal of daily activities, scheduled activities, self-reliance training, cognitive rehearsal, graded task assignments, and diversion techniques.

Indications

CBT can be used to reduce psychological distress or symptoms of a mental illness as isolated treatment. It can also be combined with medication to change beliefs that enable the development of disorders, put attention on psychosocial factors, minimize the chance of relapse after remission of illness has occurred, and increase the compliance to treatment.

Interpersonal Therapy

Interpersonal therapy (IPT) is a type of psychotherapy that is focused on the improvement of interpersonal relationships. Interpersonal therapy is useful for the treatment of depression and potentially for other conditions such as personality disorders and bulimia.

During this psychotherapy, the therapist focuses their attention on issues that arise in the present. The therapist helps patients discover problems that may affect their self-confidence and interpersonal relationships. The four domains of IPT focus are interpersonal deficits, role transitions, grief, and interpersonal disputes. After successful identification, the patient is ready to learn new adaptive behaviors and better communication strategies. ITP is done weekly for three or four months.

Supportive Psychotherapy

Supportive psychotherapy is a type of individual psychotherapy that is used to help patients through difficult times and situations. The therapist who conducts supportive psychotherapy should express concern, sympathy, and interest. Patients can talk about all the problems they experience. They may range from issues in their marriage to persecutory delusions caused by psychosis. Supportive psychotherapy can be used in all mental disorders which include psychoses and dementia.

The main aim of supportive therapy is to enable the patient to cope with difficult experiences, periods of adjustment, and other situations. The patient talks about their problem and the therapist offers advice. The therapist may teach the patient specific coping techniques such as new skills, new hobbies for their daily routine, new people, a move from their parent's home to achieve autonomy, etc. Alcoholic patients who have stopped drinking may receive words of encouragement and suggestions on how to increase self-control. This may include how to spend their free time with new sports or hobbies. Sessions should be adapted to the needs of individual patients.

Group Therapy

Group therapy is done with a large number of patients. It provides a supportive social environment that enables them to improve the ways they interact with others. Group therapy types vary. They depend on the people who comprise the group, the issues to be worked on, the settings in which they meet, the therapeutic goals, and the role the group leader takes.

Group therapy in the inpatient psychiatric setting is guided by a physician, a social worker, and a group. These groups can be composed of patients with the same disorders. For example, there can be groups for people with eating disorders or for people with psychotic disorders. Group therapy provides patients with a safe and secure environment where they can share their problems, reduce feelings of loneliness and isolation, and learn new coping skills. Group therapy can also help patients improve their social skills. Inpatient groups are usually followed by outpatient or aftercare groups. They are used to follow-up with patients and consolidate the skills they have learned in the inpatient setting.

Chapter 12: Complementary Interventions

The gold standard of care in psychiatry is psychopharmacologic and psychotherapeutic treatment. However, many people choose complementary and alternative therapies. These are considered holistic healthcare. Patients may choose complementary interventions to have more control in the decision-making process, limited insurance coverage for conventional treatment, preference for the natural, high cost of healthcare services and medications, and side-effects or failure of medications.

Complementary interventions are defined as non-conventional treatments added to conventional medical treatment. Alternative interventions are defined as non-conventional treatments given instead of conventional medical treatment. Integrative methods combine both conventional and non-conventional treatment. Complementary interventions can be categorized as natural, biologically based treatments (e.g., vitamins, supplements, and herbal products), mind and body interventions (e.g., yoga and meditation), and whole systems and body-based therapies (e.g., massage, Ayurvedic medicine, acupressure and acupuncture, reflexology).

Biologically Based Treatments

Vitamins and Dietary Supplements

Docosahexaenoic acid (DHA) is an omega-3 polyunsaturated fatty acid. It can be used for attention-deficit/hyperactivity disorder (ADHD), dyslexia, cognitive impairment, and dementia. It can also be useful as a complementary medicine for patients with depression who are on a conventional antidepressant. However, it is not used as monotherapy for depression. Adverse effects consist of anticoagulant properties and mild gastrointestinal distress. It interacts with warfarin (Coumadin) and increases the risk of bleeding. DHA should be used with caution in patients who have a risk of bleeding (e.g., patients with hemophilia or patients on anticoagulant medication). Patients should be instructed to stop using the supplement before surgery.

Choline can be used in patients with manic conditions, tardive dyskinesia, cancer, and cognitive disorders. Choline is needed for the structure and function of all cells and is beneficial for fetal brain development. It is given in doses of 300-1200mg. Higher doses (above three grams) are associated with a fishy body odor. Adverse effects include sweating, hypotension, and depression. Choline should be restricted in patients with primary genetic trimethylaminuria. It interacts with methotrexate.

5-Hydroxytryptophan (5-HTP) is an immediate precursor of serotonin. It is useful in depression, obesity, fibromyalgia, and headaches. Patients with carcinoid tumors or those who take MAOIs have a risk of serotonin syndrome with 5-HTP. There are interactions with SSRIs, MAOIs, methyldopa, St. John's wort, phenoxybenzamine, 5-HT antagonists, and 5-HT receptor agonists. The dosage ranges from 100mg to two grams daily. Its safety increases when combined with carbidopa.

The vitamin E family is an essential fat-soluble vitamin family made of tocopherols and tocotrienols. Vitamin E has immune-enhancing, antioxidant, and neuroprotective properties. It is used in neurologic disorders, diabetes, and premenstrual syndrome. It may alleviate symptoms of depression, irritability, and weight gain in patients with PMS. Vitamin E can increase the risk of bleeding in patients. It also increases the risk of hemorrhagic stroke and thrombophlebitis. Vitamin E interacts with warfarin, antiplatelet drugs (e.g., aspirin), and neomycin. Due to the increased risk of bleeding, vitamin E should be stopped before surgical procedures.

Melatonin occurs naturally in the body. It is a hormone produced by the pineal gland that regulates the circadian rhythm and sleep. It can be used for insomnia, sleep disturbances, and jet lag. Adverse effects of melatonin include the inhibition of ovulation in higher doses (1g), grogginess, depression, headache, and amnesia. Melatonin interacts with aspirin, NSAIDs, beta-blockers, sedating drugs, corticosteroids, valerian root, 5-HTP, and alcohol. It should be given in 0.3-3mg doses for short periods.

Herbal Medicine

St. John's wort (*Hypericum*) is effective for the treatment of major depressive disorders, anxiety, and sleep problems. It contains hypericin, flavonoids, and xanthones. Adverse effects include headaches, photosensitivity, and constipation. St. John's wort should not be used with SSRIs or MAOIs. There is a risk of serotonin syndrome and reports of mania when combined with sertraline (Zoloft). It should not be used with alcohol and opioids. Patients should be instructed to discontinue St. John's wort five days before surgery.

Valerian (*L.Valeriana officinalis*) contains valepotriates, valerenic acid, and caffeic acid. It is used as a sedative, muscle relaxant, and hypnotic. Valerian can cause cognitive and motor impairment, gastrointestinal upset, and hepatotoxicity. Long-term use is associated with contact allergy, headaches, restlessness, insomnia, mydriasis, and cardiac dysfunction. Valerian should not be used with alcohol or CNS depressants due to its sedative effects.

Gingko (*L. Gingko biloba*) contains flavonoids, and ginkgolide A, B. The benefits of gingko include symptomatic relief of delirium and dementia and improved concentration and memory. Gingko is a possible antidote to sexual dysfunction caused by SSRIs. Adverse effects include allergic skin reactions, gastrointestinal upset, muscle spasms, and headaches. Gingko has possible interactions with anticoagulants and increases the risk of bleeding.

Ginseng (*L.Panax ginseng*) contains triterpenes and ginsenosides. Ginseng has stimulating and mood-elevating properties. Ginseng causes insomnia, hypertonia, and edema (also called ginseng abuse syndrome). Ginseng should not be used with sedatives, hypnotic agents, MAOIs, antidiabetic agents, or steroids. Due to its anticoagulant action, it should be discontinued seven days before surgery.

Kava kava (*L.Piperismethysticum)* contains kava lactones and kava pyrone. It is used as a sedative, hypnotic, and antispasmodic. It can cause lethargy, impaired cognition, and dermatitis in patients who use it long-term. Kava kava is synergistic with anxiolytics and alcohol. Kava kava should be avoided in patients who are treated with levodopa and other dopaminergic agents. It is contraindicated in patients with endogenous depression since it can increase the danger of suicide.

Lavender (*L.Lavandula angustifolia)* contains hydroxycoumarin, tannins, and caffeic acid. It is used for its sedative and hypnotic properties. Essential oils from lavender are used in aromatherapy to treat anxiety. Adverse effects include headache, nausea, and confusion. Lavender is synergistic with other sedatives. The dosage is three to five grams per day. Lavender can cause severe toxicity but is not commonly associated with death by overdose.

How to Maintain Patient Safety and Optimize Patient's Response to Treatment

Regulation of natural supplements by the US Food and Drug Administration is not as strict as it is with traditional medications. Patients can run into misinformation on the internet. There may be a lot of variability in the purity of products. Therefore, the psychiatric mental health nurse practitioner should aim to inform patients of the pros and cons of using natural products as a part of their care. Often, patients fail to inform the healthcare provider of the use of alternative treatments. Herb-drug interactions can influence the response and tolerability of the prescribed treatment. Providers should regularly ask patients about the use of natural products and discuss their safety.

The nurse practitioner should do a full comprehensive evaluation of all-natural products and medications that patients use. Optimization can be achieved only by consideration of products that are evidence-based and have a logical mechanism of action, products that have a high benefit-to-risk ratio, and products with a defined dosage and time frame that allows for evaluation of their effects. Patients who benefit the most from natural products or supplements are those with a preference for natural products, those who have too many intolerable adverse effects from medications, and patients with inadequate nutrient intake.

Mind and Body Interventions

Exercise

Exercise is beneficial for physical and mental health. It improves overall quality of life, reduces morbidities, and improves immune system function. Exercise can reduce symptoms of depression, anxiety, and PTSD. It also improves cognitive function and self-esteem. Exercise increases the secretion of neurotransmitters such as serotonin, adrenaline, and endogenous opiates.

People with serious mental illnesses are more likely to have comorbid medical conditions. Exercise can help them improve hypertension, obesity, and diabetes. In patients with schizophrenia, exercise can reduce body mass index, improve aerobic fitness, raise self-esteem, and reduce psychiatric symptoms. It can also correct the weight gain caused by antipsychotics and improve treatment adherence.

Meditation

The goal of meditation is to enter a state of nonjudgmental attention to the present moment and awareness of sensations, feelings, sounds, and thoughts that occur in that moment. Meditation causes a sense of inner calm and has been shown to be beneficial in the treatment of many psychiatric disorders.

Mindfulness practices include mindfulness-based stress reduction (MBSR) and mindfulness-based cognitive therapy (MBCT). These programs aim to teach patients how to cultivate mindfulness and incorporate it into their daily lives. Patients are taught how to self-regulate their attention and bring it to the present moment. They also learn how to be open and accepting towards their own experience. This leads to increased cognitive flexibility and reduced repetitive negative thinking. Mindfulness practices are effective in the treatment of depressive symptoms and prevention of depression relapse. They also reduce symptoms and provide support for psychiatric issues such as eating disorders, anxiety disorders, bipolar disorders, and substance use disorders.

Mindfulness-informed interventions include dialectical behavioral therapy (DBT) and acceptance and commitment therapy (ACT). These programs incorporate mindfulness as a part of a wider treatment program. DBT was developed for patients with borderline personality disorder who are at a high risk of suicide. In DBT, mindfulness is a core skill. Patients are taught to develop mindfulness skills not just with meditation, but with use of non-meditation-based techniques and skills. These include observation, description, participation, and withholding of judgment. ACT uses mindfulness strategies with the aim to increase the patient's contact with the present moment and reduce rumination about past events and worries about future events.

Yoga

Yoga has been practiced as a means of healing and spiritual development for over 4,000 years in Eastern cultures. Western medicine now recognizes its potential as a treatment for a variety of mental disorders. The focus is the practice of Hatha Yoga and the asanas (postures). Asanas should be done slowly in order to relax and de-stress. Yoga modulates the autonomic nervous system by reducing sympathetic tone. It activates antagonistic neuromuscular systems and stimulates the limbic system.

Yoga has shown benefits in the treatment of depression, anxiety disorders, schizophrenia, somatoform disorders, addiction, mild cognitive impairment, and obsessive-compulsive disorder. It can be used as a complementary treatment for many psychiatric disorders. Yoga is generally a safe practice, but it can have side effects if not practiced correctly.

Body-Based Treatments

Aromatherapy

Aromatherapy is based on the psychological benefits associated with the essential oils of plants. Aromatic substances can be inhaled with aromatizers. Aromatherapy massage is a type of massage through which essential oils can be absorbed through the skin. Essential oils have psychological, antimicrobial, and analgesic therapeutic effects. For example, the smell of lavender can promote sleep. Aromatherapy can decrease stress and anxiety. It can also provide relief for gastrointestinal and musculoskeletal disorders. In psychotherapy, olfactory stimulation can be used to elicit positive memories and emotions.

Acupressure and Acupuncture

Acupressure and acupuncture are healing techniques used in traditional Chinese medicine. They are based on the belief that there is vital energy (chi) that flows through specific paths (meridians) that have 350 major points (acupoints). Manipulation of acupoints can correct imbalances through stimulation of energy flow or removal of energy flow blockades.

During acupressure, the acupoints are manipulated with fingers. In acupuncture, tiny needles made of sterilized silver or gold are placed into the skin. They can be left in place or manipulated by hand or with electrical stimulation to correct imbalances or blockades of energy flow. Western medicine explains that the mechanism behind acupressure and acupuncture is due to the release of endogenous neurotransmitters, endorphins, and enkephalins by nerve stimulation. These techniques have provided benefits for many conditions such as pain management, osteoarthritis, fibromyalgia, postoperative nausea and vomiting, and headaches. Psychiatric conditions that can benefit from acupressure and acupuncture include insomnia, anxiety, depression, and substance abuse.

Reflexology

Reflexology is the gentle massage of the ears, hands, and feet to stimulate the body's healing power. Reflexology is thought to clear crystalline deposits that are found under the skin which may interfere with the flow of the body's energy. According to reflexologists, applying pressure to an area that represents a body part can cause relief from illness in the represented body part.

Chapter 13: Care Coordination

Care coordination is a process that helps patients with mental health issues receive the best possible care and achieve the best outcome. It can be defined as a deliberate organization of the activities in patient care among healthcare professionals. Healthcare providers interact with different clinicians, patients, their family members, caretakers, and other important persons. Coordination of services can help ensure that the patient receives the right treatment at the right time.

Care coordination in mental health involves the creation of a network of mental health providers that will develop a comprehensive plan. This will help patients deal with and manage their needs. The main goal is to make sure that each unique, individual patient receives the appropriate services and support at the right time. The focus is to provide close communication and collaboration between various mental healthcare professionals. These include mental health providers, psychiatrists, psychologists, primary care providers, psychiatric mental health nurse practitioners, social workers, and community mental health centers.

Professional Communication

There are many interfaces and patient handoffs between mental healthcare practitioners in the current healthcare system. Healthcare providers have various levels of education and occupational training. A patient may interact with 50 different staff members such as nurses, psychiatrists, and technicians during a short hospital stay. All team members must have close collaboration. Accurate communication of critical information is necessary in an effective clinical practice. Miscommunications between healthcare providers can endanger patient safety due to misinterpretation, lack of critical information, unclear orders over the phone, and unnoticed changes in the patient's physical or psychiatric status.

Medical errors are a consequence of a lack of communication. Medical errors can result in injury or patient death. Communication failures are considered among the leading causes of delays in treatment and medication errors. Communication and collaboration between team members is necessary to minimize the rate of medical errors and ensure patient safety.

<u>Communication and Team Collaboration</u>

Communication is the transmission of information through writing, speech, or signs. In healthcare, important information is transferred by e-mails, text messages, or handwritten notes. Any miscommunication in healthcare can have dire consequences.

Collaboration in healthcare is achieved when healthcare providers work together cooperatively. They take on complementary roles, share responsibility, and make decisions that aid in the development of plans for patient care. Through collaboration, healthcare team members gain awareness of each other's skills and knowledge. This improves decision-making. The most effective teams are characterized by the presence of respect, collaboration, and trust.

For a successful teamwork model, an interdisciplinary approach should be implemented in healthcare. In a multidisciplinary approach, every team member takes responsibility for actions that are related to their discipline. They develop individual treatment plans for the patient. In an interdisciplinary approach, all team members from various disciplines coalesce together in a joint effort to develop a common goal for the patient.

Patients find it easier to communicate with cohesive teams compared to various professionals who are unaware of the contributions of others in the care of the patient. An integrated healthcare plan consists of multiple assessments, integrated interventions, and treatment regimens.

The most important components of successful teamwork include clear direction, open communication, clear and known roles for the members, a respectful atmosphere and compassionate environment, balance of member participation during tasks, a clear decision-making process, an enabling environment, and accessible resources. Frequent communication and sharing of information, conflict resolution skills, and appropriate mechanisms for outcome measurement are also essential. Teams must have the ability to adjust accordingly.

Certain obstacles may arise in the development of a collaborative environment. These include a perceived loss of autonomy, a clash of perceptions, additional time, and lack of confidence in others. These obstacles can be overcome through mutual respect, trust, and an open attitude. Collaboration and teamwork are among the most important factors that can improve clinical effectiveness.

Unfortunately, barriers to communication, teamwork, and collaboration can occur in the clinical setting. For example, communication failures that have resulted in adverse clinical outcomes can sometimes be attributed to social and relational structures. Different members of the same healthcare team can have different priorities for patient care. This may cause inconsistencies in verbal communication. Many patients have reported that they were not aware of who was in charge of their care during a hospital stay. They have also reported that healthcare staff provided them with conflicting information.

There can be issues related to physician and nurse disruptive behaviors that can be traced to failures in collaboration and communication. This may include inappropriate behavior, conflict, confrontation, verbal abuse, physical abuse, and sexual harassment. These issues have an impact on staff satisfaction, and patient outcomes (medical errors, preventable mortality, adverse effects, patient safety, and others).

In the healthcare setting, many professionals have come to recognize communication and teamwork failures. This has developed a culture of low expectations. In this type of culture, many medical errors can occur. Even the most diligent healthcare providers may start to ignore discrepancies and red flags. They may also expect a partial and faulty exchange of information. Effective communication can result in many positive outcomes such as effective therapeutic interventions, improved patient safety, improved patient and family satisfaction, decreased lengths of hospital stay, enhanced job satisfaction and employee morale, and improved information flow. Effective communication encourages continuous and clear patient care, fosters teamwork, and minimizes medical errors.

Handoff Communication

Handoff communication is the transfer of critical information, authority, and the duty to care for the patient between different healthcare providers. An effective handoff consists of a continuous and effective transition of essential information, care, and treatment. Inadequate handoff communication results in adverse outcomes and compromised patient safety.

Definition of Handoff

Other terms that describe handoff include cross-coverage, shift report, and sign-out. Handoff is a complex process that involves communication during changes of shifts and information tools that help healthcare providers communicate about patient care. Handoff provides essential information about the patient.

Issues of Handoff Communication

With the specialization and evolution of healthcare, the number of providers in patient care has increased. There are more handoffs in the current healthcare delivery system compared to the less complex systems of the past. Issues of handoff can result in failures of patient care, compromised patient safety, medication errors, and increased morbidity and mortality. There are many challenges for effective communication in the complex and dynamic clinical setting. With technological advancements and increased specialization in healthcare, all providers need to address the issues associated with fragmented care and ineffective handoffs.

An example of an ineffective handoff is the use of sign-out sheets. Doctors frequently use sign-out sheets for communication. However, sign-out sheets are associated with mistakes such as missing allergies, incorrect weight, and errors in medication information.

Another issue is contact with the correct healthcare provider in the organizationally complex acute care hospitals. The complex organization and increased number of specialties and physicians that provide care to one patient contribute to difficulties in communication. Many physicians have reported that they are often unable to identify the primary nurse who is responsible for the patient. Many nurses have had trouble with the identification of the primary physician in charge of the patient.

Effective handoff depends on the knowledge, experience level, and interpersonal communication skills of the healthcare provider. There is an issue with the transition of care among healthcare providers because of an educational gap. Many medical schools and nursing programs do not teach how to effectively handoff patients. Doctors and nurses have different patterns of communication. Nurses may give broader descriptions of situations. Physicians tend to focus on critical information bullets. The SBAR (situation, background, assessment, recommendation) briefing model is one technique that aims to improve handoff communication. It intends to bridge the communication style gap between doctors and nurses.

Where Handoffs Occur

Handoffs can occur in all types of healthcare settings. There are a variety of handoffs between healthcare providers. These include the transitions of essential information and responsibility of care during the handoff between shifts or the transfer of the patient from one unit to another in the same hospital.

When the transfer occurs between nurses and physicians or nurses and diagnostic personnel, the handoff is called interdisciplinary. When the handoff occurs between physicians or between nurses, the handoff is called intradisciplinary. When handoffs occur between hospitals and organizations such as extended-care facilities or home health agencies, the handoffs are called interfacility handoffs.

Specialized technology such as computerized records, handheld devices, pagers, audio records, or written documents can be used in the handoff process. There are unique challenges that come with different types and locations of handoff.

Shift-to-Shift Handoff

Many human factors influence the handoff process during shift changes. During shift-to-shift handoff, healthcare providers have a responsibility to ensure patient safety. They transmit important patient care information, promote continuous patient care, and ensure that the patient is transferred to a competent and qualified nurse. The organizational culture of the clinical setting influences the intershift handoff. In a clinical setting where the staff is allowed to openly communicate and express concerns, the culture is one of safety. The shift-to-shift handoff is a complex process. If done poorly it may result in adverse patient outcomes.

Method of Shift-to-Shift Handoff

Methods that are used in shift-to-shift handoff include handwritten notes, electronic reports, verbal communication, bedside reports, computer printouts, audiotapes, telephones, and memory. All these methods have strengths and weaknesses.

The verbal report on the nursing unit can provide an educational opportunity for the staff and allow face-to-face interactions. It is convenient for clarification of information and to debrief and discuss situations. The downsides are that the receiver may not retain information because the report is verbal only. It can be time-consuming and cause sensory overload. To reduce the loss of information, an augmented verbal report can be used with preprinted forms that contain data about the specific patient. With the use of electronic support, the staff can have easy access to accurate and up-to-date data.

A verbal report at the patient's bedside has certain strengths. These include patient involvement, face-to-face interaction, and ability to clarify information. However, it presents confidentiality issues and issues related to the use of technical jargon by nurses. Not every patient wants to participate in the bedside report. These obstacles can be overcome through introduction of the nurses, encouragement of patients to participate, monitoring to ensure protected confidentiality, and use of a developed protocol that will guide the handover process.

The audiotaped report is efficient, concise, and less time-consuming. Nurses can repeat the tape to understand the information better. While the nurses from the oncoming shift listen to the audiotaped report, the nurses who recorded the report can provide patient care. The audiotaped report has some weaknesses. These include difficulty in comprehension, sensory overload, lack of educational opportunity, the need for access to equipment, and potential discrepancies between the actual patient status and reported patient status. The tape may not be recorded in the current timeline. To improve the audiotaped report, the sound quality should be ensured. There should be an interaction between the offgoing and ongoing shift in to ensure opportunities for questions about the report. Bedside rounds should be included to check the congruence of the patient's status between the report and their actual condition.

The written report allows the oncoming shift to make review of essential data. It allows effective management and represents a documentation improvement. The weaknesses of the written report include variations in the quality of documentation, the absence of question-and-answer interaction, and the potential to miss essential information if not documented. Weaknesses can be overcome through interactions between the offgoing and ongoing shifts. The offgoing shift should provide verbal information along with the written report. A standardized process should be used to ensure that essential information is conveyed.

Chapter 14: Therapeutic Environment Management

The therapeutic environment is an especially important factor that plays a role in the management of patients with mental health issues. When the patient comes into the hospital or any other space, the environment is the first thing they encounter. The therapeutic environment will affect how the person experiences initial and subsequent meetings.

The therapeutic environment should be a place of acceptance, positive regard, and empathetic understanding. In this environment, patients should feel as if they can verbalize their thoughts freely and express their behaviors and emotions without judgment. Patients should feel that they can make constructive changes to their reactions and attitudes to improve their quality of life. The experience of a patient as they enter a therapeutic environment should be beneficial and pleasant.

What is a Therapeutic Environment?

A therapeutic environment is where a person who suffers from mental health issues will find it easy to talk about sensitive and potentially disturbing topics such as trauma. A therapeutic environment elicits an unconscious sense of safety in people. This reduces their defenses and resistance. The healthcare staff must make a conscious effort to create a therapeutic environment.

In construction of a therapeutic environment, the healthcare staff can further progress to other milestones. These include treatment goals, personal growth, and a positive impact in the lives of people who seek mental health services. The psychiatric mental health nurse practitioner should consider various aspects of the environment such as interpersonal and intrapersonal boundaries, engagement, communication, physical space, and safety (emotional, environmental, and physical).

Safety is number one on the list of considerations for a therapeutic environment. A simple way to assess this is to ascertain your own feelings of safety in the environment and what you can do to increase the sense of safety. The room where the patient will be seen should also give a sense of comfort. Patients who feel uncomfortable will find it hard to engage during therapy. Other aspects that should not be overlooked include engagement and communication. The nurse should be aware that engagement and communication skills can reveal whether the healthcare staff is genuinely concerned for the patient's outcome and well-being.

There are many approaches for the creation of a therapeutic environment. For example, some people consider a private and comfortable space to be essential. Psychology has played a role to shape the spaces used for therapeutic purposes. The idea that the most effective therapeutic response occurs in a home setting has resulted in the creation of intensive in-home and other home-based interventions. In home-based interventions, the services are delivered at the home of the patient. In this case, the therapist has limited control over the environment. Conventional therapy is delivered in the office of the therapist where they have the most control. The best choice depends on the individual patient and their needs.

How to Create the Therapeutic Environment

Physical and interactive spaces are two factors to be considered in the creation of a therapeutic environment. The healthcare staff invests energy, focus, planning, conscious effort, and evaluation as well as financial means to create an optimal experience for patients who seek mental health resources.

Context

Therapeutic environments exist in a wide variety of contexts. Some exist in a traditional context and others aim for an integrated health-care approach. The most commonly served populations in the therapeutic environment include patients with severe and persistent mental illness, developmental disabilities, and substance use disorder. These populations can be served in different locations where a variety of services can be provided. The mental health services should be specific to the needs of the populations that are being served. These can include residential programs, outpatient programs, day programs, etc.

Recommendations for the Structure of the Optimal Therapeutic Environment

Studies in environmental psychology have been done to determine the type of therapeutic environment that is most beneficial and pleasing for patients. These studies survey people their level of comfort in the places where they have received therapy. Many factors come into play in the structure of the environment. Therapy can be done in clinics, community spaces, facilities, homes, private practice offices, counseling centers, rehabilitation centers, and other community-based locations.

Physical Environment

People begin their experience before they enter a building. For the therapy session to be productive, the staff should make sure that people will feel a sense of safety before they enter the counseling session. The office where therapy is conducted should be away from the main road since busy streets or freeways can cause stress. This may have a negative influence on the therapeutic work. People in a crowded situation are more likely to feel anxious and stressed. The size of the parking lot should also be considered. There should be enough parking spaces for all patients and staff to feel welcome. There should be enough parking spaces for staff and visitors as well. The staff should also make sure there is enough parking access for vehicles used by people with disabilities.

Therapeutic Milieu

The therapeutic milieu is a carefully structured, specific type of environment that aims to keep patients safe and provide them with the highest number of benefits. Milieu therapy enables patients to learn new skills and encourages attitudes of respect and positivity. It supports patients on the journey towards recovery.

Milieu therapy is not limited to the support of a safe physical environment. It consists of the support of therapists, nurses, social workers, and other healthcare staff. The therapeutic milieu is seen in a variety of settings such as rehabilitation facilities, outpatient and inpatient clinics, hospitals, private therapeutic offices, and even at home. Patients who trust in the therapeutic milieu feel empowered to try new adaptive coping skills. Milieu therapy consists of a structured environment, support, consistent expectations, mutual respect, a focus on the needs of the patient, evenly distributed power, and repetition.

A Structured Environment

Entrance and Exit

The building in which therapy is conducted should be easy to identify. People should be able to locate it easily. The entrance should be free from obstruction so people know where the waiting area is. The entrance should be made accessible for patients with disabilities. For example, the building should have a ramp for entrance and exit and easy access to restrooms. If possible, the exit and waiting area should be in different locations. The receptionist should be pleasant and warm. There should be a private space for the collection of confidential data.

Privacy

The waiting area is a place between the calmness of counseling sessions and the emotionality of daily life. In the waiting area, people can collect their inner feelings and thoughts. The noise level should be brought to a minimum. You should discourage phone use in the waiting area since people might not want to overhear the conversations of others. The furniture should be comfortable and the space should be maintained and clean. Appropriate decorations, plants, books, magazines, and other reading material increase the comfort of the room.

Patients should have routines such as scheduled daily activities, individual therapy, psychosocial education, recreation therapy, mealtimes, free time, group therapy, occupational training, and art therapy. This allows patients to try out new behavioral patterns in a safe, supportive environment.

Office Design

A pleasant and well-maintained physical space should make people feel comfortable. To increase self-disclosure, the room where therapy is conducted should have a warm and intimate setting. A small room can have a negative influence on therapeutic communication. A wide room can support a healthy therapeutic alliance. However, if the room is too big, it may elicit feelings of insecurity in the patient. Office decorations can have symbolic meanings for patients. Clinicians should consider decorations that may induce a certain belief about the clinician which may cause negative or positive transference. Plants are a positive decoration since they remind patients of natural environments. Pictures of nature can also induce a calming effect.

Seating

The patient and therapist should be at an intermediate distance. This is between 48 to 60 inches. People feel a certain autonomy and increased comfort when they have control over movable furniture such as chairs or pillows. The seating arrangement can also elicit a sense of autonomy. Adults should sit in large chairs or sofas. Children should be placed in smaller chairs.

Lighting and Color

Natural light has the most beneficial effect on patients. Natural light reduces negative emotions and increases well-being. However, if natural lighting is not possible, dim or soft lighting is preferable to fluorescent lighting. Dim or soft lightning has a calming effect on patients. Lamps and indirect lightning make the atmosphere more pleasant.

Preferences of color vary across different ages and genders. However, the most practical choice for a therapy setting is neutral, soft, and light colors. The choice of color can elicit a sense of calmness for both patient and therapist.

Noise Level/Privacy

The healthcare staff should make efforts to minimize external and office noise so the therapeutic session does not get distracted. Patients feel more comfortable to fully engage in therapy when they are in soundproof rooms. White noise machines can be used to make the patient more comfortable with self-disclosure and ensure confidentiality.

Smell, Texture, and Temperature

A smell can trigger old memories and emotional or physical responses. Offices should have a neutral smell with no intense perfumes or colognes. Soft textures create a comfortable setting. The ideal temperature is around 68-72 degrees Fahrenheit (average room temperature). Patients may become distracted if they feel too hot or too cold.

Safety and Security

Establishment of safety and security is necessary for the therapy session to guide the person toward healing. Safety and security involve communication and connection with the therapist and the physical space. The relationship with the clinical provider is very important to establish safety and security. The therapeutic milieu consists of both physical and non-physical aspects of the environment. Patients in the therapeutic environment should feel safe from physical and emotional danger. A safe environment can be created through the establishment of expectations, consistency, and boundaries.

The environment should feel homelike to the patient. They should be able to express themselves without expectation or fear of rejection. Provisions of consistency and behavioral expectations allow the patient and therapist to know what to expect from each other. Vulnerability is another key factor to establish safety and security. The therapeutic milieu should be a trusting environment and allow patients to share their deepest and scariest parts. Community and group settings have the advantage to build empathy as patients are exposed to the struggles and emotions of other people.

Benefits of the Therapeutic Milieu

In the therapeutic milieu, patients will feel physically and emotionally safe, encouraged to take on responsibility for their actions, and able to try new adaptive behaviors in an environment that is safe and supportive. Patients get feedback from the therapist and other healthcare staff. This allows them to learn and improve their skills. Patients can get creative about new ideas to help them handle the difficulties of everyday life.

Chapter 15: Therapeutic Communication

Therapeutic communication is very important to facilitate a productive patient-provider relationship. Many techniques can be used to help the healthcare provider obtain necessary information. Some interventions are counterproductive and can obstruct the interview. To achieve the best outcome, the psychiatric-mental health nurse practitioner should use facilitative interventions, motivational interviewing, expanded interventions, etc.

Facilitative Interventions

Facilitative interventions enable the patient to share their own story. They can help build a positive relationship between the healthcare provider and the patient. All these techniques can be combined or they can be isolated.

Reinforcement

Reinforcement is a very useful method to get the patient to share more information about their situation. Reinforcement is achieved with simple phrases such as "I see," "Hmm," "Yes," and "Go on." These phrases show that the interviewer is interested. This encourages the patient to continue talking. They should fit naturally into the interview.

Reflection

Reflection is done through the use of the patient's words. Reflection informs the patient that the clinician has listened to what they have said, that they understand them, and want to know more. To avoid sounding robotic, you can paraphrase the patient's words.

Summary

Summary should be done during the interview to sum up what has been recognized about the topic. By summarizing, the patient gets to know what the psychiatrist's understanding of the situation is. If it's needed, the patient can clarify or add new information. If the patient adds new information, the psychiatrist might continue the previous topic and explore the new information later.

Reassurance

Reassurance for the patient is helpful. It can decrease their anxiety about the illness and encourage them to continue the discussion. It can also motivate the patient to continue treatment. Reassuring patients when the outcome is still unknown is inappropriate. When there are many unknown variables, the psychiatrist can provide reassurance that they will work together to understand and manage the situation.

Acknowledgment of Emotion

Acknowledgment of the emotion the patient expresses can enable them to share more feelings openly. Nonverbal actions such as placement of the tissue box closer to the patient can be helpful in this regard if used appropriately. If the patient is clearly expressing an emotion, such as openly crying, then it is better to comment on the associated feelings rather than the direct emotion.

Humor

Sometimes patients like to tell jokes. Smiling or laughing at the joke can be helpful in this situation. Humor decreases anxiety and adds a genuine feeling to the interview atmosphere. The clinician should be sure that the patient intended to make a funny comment and that they laugh at the joke, not at the patient.

Silence

Silence, when used appropriately, can progress the interview. During the interview, the patient may need to experience an emotion or to think about what was said. If the psychiatrist's anxiety ends the silence prematurely, that may hinder the patient's insight or expression of feeling. However, too many periods of silence can also negatively affect the interview. The patient might get bored and look at their watch or around the room. In this situation, you can comment, "It looks to me like you're thinking about other things."

Obstructive Interventions

Obstructive interventions disrupt the development of a positive provider-patient relationship. Facilitating interventions can become obstructive if they are unclear, used at an inappropriate time, not responsive to the patient's issues, and unconnected. Obstructive interventions can also be called "roadblocks to active listening."

Closed-Ended Questions

Closed-ended questions can halt the progression of the patient's story. Patients can come prepared for therapy, especially if they have previous experience. They are ready to talk about painful topics. If the psychiatrist avoids blocking the patient with too many closed-ended questions, the patient can be a partner in the interview. Psychiatrists learn to redefine their skills during the interview.

Judgmental Questions or Statements

Judgmental interventions stop the patient from being open about sensitive or intimate information. Judgment is nonproductive and can obstruct the development of a respectful relationship. Criticism, disagreement, and blame can make the patient feel as if something is wrong with them. Sometimes patients can interpret a simple disagreement as critical. It may be more useful to ask the patient if they think their actions lead to productive results.

Minimization of Patient's Concerns

Sometimes the therapist might minimize the patient's concern in an attempt to reassure them. In this situation, the patient might feel as if the therapist does not truly understand their suffering. Exploration of the concern can lead to the discovery of new information that may be relevant to the treatment plan.

Nonverbal Communication

The importance of nonverbal communication should not be underestimated. A therapist who looks at their watch, yawns, looks at the computer screen, or turns away from the patient may seem disinterested or bored. This might make the patient feel unimportant. These types of actions can ruin the relationship between the provider and the patient.

Premature Interpretation and Advice

A patient might feel misunderstood and act defensively when the therapist makes premature interpretations. This can happen even when the interpretation is correct. Premature advice is ineffective because early in the interview the therapist does not know all of the factors at play. This might obstruct the patient's wish to create a plan for themselves.

Intense Questioning

Intense questioning can be mistaken for good listening. You might want to ask more questions to get to know the patient better but this might make the patient feel as if they are being interrogated. Often, too many questions do not lead to the right answer.

Motivational Interviewing

Many mental health conditions require a behavioral change to achieve the best clinical outcome. The absence of a behavioral change might be a reason for poor outcomes in some patients. In these situations, it is useful to inspire the patient to collaborate and participate actively in their journey to health. Patients may respond better to a family-centered model that uses motivational interviewing rather than a disciplinary expert-providing advice approach.

Motivational interviewing is a client-centered method that aims to increase the patient's inner motivation for change through resolve of their ambivalence. Motivational interviewing meets patients at the level of their problem recognition. It is useful for patients who are treated for psychoactive substance abuse, smoking cessation, reduction of HIV-risk behaviors, eating disorders, and poor medication compliance. It is also useful in patients who are high in ambivalence (they have mixed feelings about change), patients with low self-confidence who doubt they have the capabilities to change, patients who have a low desire to change, and patients who are unaware of the advantages of change. It is important to remember that with motivational interviewing the nurse practitioner treats the patient as an equal. Nurses should refrain from giving unsolicited advice, warnings, instructions, and confrontations.

Core Skills of Motivational Interviewing (OARS)

Motivational interviewing consists of four core counseling skills that can be remembered with the acronym O (Open questions), A (Affirming), R (Reflective listening), S (Summarizing).

Open Questions

Open questions enable patients to tell their stories. Closed questions are used to gather brief information. With an open question, you give the patient a chance to reflect and elaborate before answering. Their answers will help you understand things from their perspective. Open questions start dialogues and do not require a specific answer from the psychiatric mental health nurse practitioner. The patient feels encouraged to do most of the talking. Closed questions can make patients feel as if they need to have the right answer.

Affirming

Affirming is a way to show the patient you have a positive regard for them and genuinely appreciate them. Affirming increases the patient's self-confidence and encourages them to take action. Affirming should not be confused with praise. When affirming, you should highlight the patient's present efforts and strengths, as well as their past successes. The statements should be more focused on the patient with use of "you" instead of "I." For example, "You are working hard to improve your life and make a positive change." Other examples of affirmations include, "You are taking a big step by participating in this treatment," or "You are trying hard to avoid situations that might cause you to drink."

Reflective Listening

Reflective listening expresses empathy through respect and acceptance of patients, establishment of trust, nonjudgmental relationship, and encouragement to explore emotions, values, and perceptions. Reflective listening allows the psychiatric mental health nurse practitioner to show support without consistent agreement with the patient. Reflective listening is a tool that reinforces change. It shows that you want to understand the patient's perspective and feelings. Differences in culture and ethnicity might impact how the patient and the nurse interpret nonverbal and verbal communication.

Reflective listening requires the healthcare provider to actively listen to the patient, make a hypothesis about the meaning or emotion of the patient's statement, and reflect the best guess back to the patient. There are several types of reflective listening. Simple reflective listening consists of repetition or rephrasing of statements. It shows the patient that you want to understand their perspective. Complex reflective listening consists of reflecting the underlying meaning of a statement. This encourages patients to deeply explore themselves.

Simple reflections are less challenging than complex reflections. They only require you to repeat or rephrase what the patient has said. Complex reflections require a mental hypothesis about what the patient has said. For example, if the patient says, "I drink because I feel alone," it's important to consider what they mean. A reflective listening response would be, "You drink because it is hard for you to find friends." The patient's verbal or nonverbal response will inform you if you are on the right track. If the patient elaborates on the initial statement, it means your guess was probably correct.

The basis of reflective listening is to make a mental hypothesis and then express your hypothesis with a reflective statement. Observe the patient's response to check if your hypothesis is correct. Ideally, you should follow up with an open question after two or three reflective listening responses. Reflective listening helps build a strong relationship with the patient and facilitates their self-exploration. These are two main components of client-centered counseling.

Summarizing

Summarizing is a type of reflective listening that aims to present a full picture of the patient's experience with a few statements that have meaning and reflect them to the patient. Motivational interviewing identifies several types of summarizing. These include:

- Collecting summary (creates a narrative).
- Linking summary (reflects a statement and links it to an earlier one).
- Transitional summary (progresses the change process).
- Ambivalence summary.
- Recapitulation summary (summarizes the talk about change and helps create a new change plan).

When the summary ends, you should ask the patient if they have something more to add. This encourages self-reflection.

Chapter 16: Medication Management

Psychopharmacology is the mainstay of care in modern psychiatry. Psychopharmacology enables the patient to achieve a neurochemical homeostasis which then can be used as a productive environment in which they can learn adaptive coping mechanisms. The psychiatric-mental health nurse practitioner must be educated on the pharmacology of psychiatric medications. This chapter will explain the basic pharmacological principles (e.g., pharmacokinetics and pharmacodynamics), the optimization of pharmacological treatment to achieve the best clinical outcome, and potential adverse effects.

Drug Factors

How an individual patient will respond to a drug depends on genetic and environmental factors. Drugs that are effective in some patients may not be effective in others. Drugs vary from each other by differences in their molecular structure, interactions with neurotransmitters, pharmacokinetics, protein binding, and the presence of active metabolites. Drug factors and patient factors influence the efficacy, tolerability, and safety of treatment. A good understanding of these factors increases the chance of successful treatment.

Pharmacokinetics

Pharmacokinetics is defined as *what the body does to the drug*. Pharmacokinetic principles include absorption, distribution, metabolism, and elimination. Absorption is the journey of the drug through the bloodstream from the site of administration. Distribution is the movement of the drug from the bloodstream to the organs. The blood flow and protein content of organs influence distribution. The free unbound portion of the drug is the active part while the protein-bound is inactive. Patients who have low protein levels (e.g., patients with anorexia nervosa) are at risk of increased toxicity due to the increased unbound portion of the drug.

Metabolism is the chemical alteration of the drug or breakdown before elimination. First-pass metabolism refers to the metabolization of drugs by the cytochrome P450 enzymes in the liver and in the intestines before reaching systemic circulation. Cytochrome P450 inducers increase the metabolism and decrease the therapeutic concentration of drugs. They include carbamazepine, St. John's wort, phenytoin, phenobarbital, and tobacco.

Cytochrome P450 inhibitors decrease the metabolism and increase the therapeutic concentration of the drugs. They include bupropion, clomipramine, cimetidine, clarithromycin, fluoroquinolones, grapefruit, ketoconazole, nefazodone, and SSRIs.

Elimination refers to the removal of the drug from the body. Factors that influence pharmacokinetics include age (young children are fast metabolizers, and therefore have lower concentrations of drugs, while elderly patients are slow metabolizers, and therefore have higher concentrations of drugs and increased chance of toxicity), race (due to genetic variations), physiological integrity (e.g., liver disease or renal insufficiency), nutritional status, and intracellular volume.

Pharmacodynamics

Pharmacodynamics refers to *what the drug does to the body.* Pharmacodynamic principles include the drug's mechanism of action, therapeutic index, dose-response curve, receptors, tolerance, withdrawal, and dependence.

Receptors are the target sites for the drugs. When drugs bind to a receptor, they can exert an agonistic effect (activate a biological response), inverse agonistic effect (reduce the activity of the receptor below its basal level by binding to the same receptor), partial agonistic effect (partially activate the receptors), or antagonistic effect (bind to the receptor without activating it).

Some drugs are enzyme inhibitors. These stop or slow down a catalytic enzyme's reaction, which allows the neurotransmitter to remain in the synaptic cleft. Monoamine oxidase inhibitors inhibit the breakdown of serotonin, dopamine, and norepinephrine.

Reuptake inhibitors block carrier proteins or reuptake pumps responsible for the reuptake of neurotransmitters back to the presynaptic neuron. This increases the concentration of neurotransmitters in the synaptic cleft. For example, selective serotonin reuptake inhibitors block the reuptake of serotonin.

Pharmacological Management

The first step in the pharmacological management process is to identify the main symptoms and proceed with making a diagnosis. The use of relevant screening tools can assist in the diagnostic process. The illness can be in its acute or chronic phase, or it can be a relapse or recurrence. Identifying the phase of the illness has implications for treatment. Personal and family history of response to medications should be recorded to identify positive or adverse responses. The patient's motivations about treatment should be assessed as well as any potential doubts or fears. A medication review should be performed to identify potential interactions between prescribed medications (including over-the-counter drugs and supplements).

The psychiatric mental health nurse practitioner should inform the patient of the risks and benefits of a medication, as well as document informed consent. The patient should have an understanding of the target symptoms, benefits, adverse effects, risks, potential comorbid complications, and potential alternatives to treatment. Patients should be informed that certain illnesses such as bipolar disorder, schizophrenia, anxiety disorders, and refractory depression may require lifelong treatment.

During treatment, the PMHNP should monitor for comorbidity, response to treatment, and serious adverse effects. Standardized clinical rating scales can determine the patient's baseline when starting treatment, and they can be used to monitor the patient's progress or decompensation throughout treatment. Before starting treatment, you should check hepatic and renal function, hemoglobin A1C, thyroid function, and lipids, and perform an EKG to check for QT prolongation.

The PMNHNP should assist in determining the length of treatment, as well as plan for potential relapse. There is a large body of evidence-based data that supports the use of combined pharmacologic and nonpharmacologic treatment in psychiatry. Patients should be offered the possibility of combined treatment to obtain the best clinical outcomes. Nonadherence to treatment should be considered since this can be a common problem in all illnesses. The patient should be asked about their smoking status since tobacco products are CYP450 inducers, and that can influence the dose of some medications.

Adverse Effects

Adverse effects are unavoidable when starting treatment with any medication. Prescribing clinicians should be aware of the more common adverse effects, and those with serious medical risks. When prescribing, you should consider the side effect's impact on the patient's quality of life, its cause, and its time course. Even the most common side effects do not occur in every patient.

Based on their time course, adverse effects can be categorized as early-onset, late-appearing, persistent, and time-limited. Nausea occurs as an early-onset, time-limited side effect when starting treatment with SSRIs or venlafaxine. An example of a late-appearing side effect is weight gain with antidepressant treatment.

Adverse effects may cause drug discontinuation. Some adverse effects are intolerable and cause a severe impact on the patient's quality of life. Serious side effects with medical consequences include agranulocytosis (clozapine), hepatic failure (nefazodone), heart block (thioridazine), stroke (phenelzine), and Stevens-Johnson syndrome (lamotrigine). Antipsychotics cause a prolongation in the QTc interval and may worsen the syndrome of inappropriate antidiuretic hormone (SIADH). Treatment with clozapine should be registered in the Risk Evaluation and Mitigation Strategies (REMS) database. Drugs that carry a risk of life-threatening consequences must be closely monitored.

Medication-Induced Movement Disorders

Medication-induced movement disorders are most commonly associated with first-generation antipsychotics (FGAs) and drugs used to treat psychosis (DRAs). The mechanism behind the abnormal motor activity is the blockade of dopamine type 2 (D2) receptors. Since SGAs block dopamine receptors to a lesser extent than first-generation antipsychotics, they are less likely to cause movement disorders.

Neuroleptic-Induced Parkinsonism

Signs and symptoms of neuroleptic-induced Parkinsonism include muscle stiffness (lead pipe rigidity), cogwheel rigidity, stooped posture, drooling, coarse tremors, tremors of the lips and perioral muscles (rabbit syndrome), and shuffling gait. Parkinsonian side effects usually occur five to ninety days after starting treatment, and most commonly affect the elderly and female patients. High-potency drugs with low anticholinergic activity, such as haloperidol, have a higher risk of causing medication-induced Parkinsonism. Treatment consists of anticholinergic agents such as benztropine, amantadine, or diphenhydramine.

Neuroleptic Malignant Syndrome

Neuroleptic malignant syndrome is a rare, potentially life-threatening complication that may occur during treatment with antipsychotics. It presents with muscular rigidity, dystonia, mutism, akinesia, obtundation, agitation, hyperthermia, increased pulse and blood pressure, and diaphoresis. Laboratory examination shows an elevated white blood cell count, and increased creatinine phosphokinase, plasma myoglobin, liver enzymes, and myoglobinuria. The symptoms of neuroleptic malignant syndrome can last from ten to fourteen days if left untreated. The diagnosis can be missed since the withdrawal or increased agitation may mimic the exacerbation of psychosis. Treatment consists of supportive medical treatment and medications such as dantrolene, bromocriptine, and amantadine. The antipsychotic dose should be as low as possible. High-potency drugs have the highest risk of inducing neuroleptic-malignant syndrome.

Medication-Induced Acute Dystonia

Dystonia is defined as prolonged muscle contractions that cause abnormal movements or postures. Dystonia presents as oculogyric crises, protrusions of the tongue, laryngeal-pharyngeal dystonias, dystonic postures of the limbs and trunk, trismus, blepharospasm, and glossopharyngeal dystonia. Dystonia most commonly affects men, patients younger than thirty years, and patients who are on high-potency antipsychotics. Treatment consists of intramuscular anticholinergics or intravenous/intramuscular diphenhydramine. Other effective treatments include diazepam, amobarbital, caffeine sodium benzoate, and hypnosis.

Medication-Induced Acute Akathisia

The definition of akathisia includes a subjective feeling of restlessness or objective visible signs of restlessness. Patients complain of a sense of anxiety and inability to relax. On examination, they present with jitteriness, rocking motions while sitting, pacing back and forth, and alterations between sitting and standing. Medications associated with akathisia include antipsychotics, sympathomimetics, and antidepressants. Middle-aged women have the highest risk of akathisia. Treatment consists of reduction of the medication to the lowest effective dose possible and beta-adrenergic receptor antagonists. Other effective medications include anticholinergic drugs, benzodiazepines, and cyproheptadine.

Tardive Dyskinesia

Tardive dyskinesia is a late-appearing side effect of antipsychotics. The patient presents with abnormal, choreoathetoid movements that affect the muscles of the head, extremities, and trunk with variable severity. The most commonly affected area is the perioral area and includes twisting and protruding movements of the tongue, lip-puckering, grimaces in the face, and chewing and lateral jaw movements. Severe cases may present with torticollis, retrocollis, trunk twisting, pelvic thrusting, respiratory dyskinesia, and breathing and swallowing irregularities. The disorder remits in most mild cases. The development of tardive dyskinesia can be prevented by using antipsychotics in the lowest effective doses only when indicated. SGAs are associated with less tardive dyskinesia. Clozapine has the least risk of tardive dyskinesia and may even be used to improve symptoms of tardive dyskinesia due to its low D2 receptor affinity and high 5-HT receptor antagonism. The Abnormal Involuntary Movement Scale (AIMS) examination procedure is used to detect abnormal movements.

Adverse Effects Associated with New Medications

Somnolence

When treating insomnia, anxiety, and agitation, the aim is to induce sedation with psychotropic drugs. However, daytime sleepiness, or somnolence, can occur as an unwanted side effect. Somnolence can impair the quality of life of patients and may endanger the safety of patients who operate vehicles or any type of mechanical equipment. SSRIs may cause somnolence due to impaired sleep quality. Patients who are on chronic treatment with SSRIs may experience fatigue or exhaustion despite getting adequate amounts of sleep. Somnolence can be managed by adjusting the dosage or timing of administration, or with the addition of small doses of stimulants or modafinil. The clinician can also consider switching to an alternative medication that does not cause somnolence.

Gastrointestinal Disturbances

Older antidepressants and antipsychotics have significant gastrointestinal side effects, such as constipation, due to their anticholinergic activity. Newer drugs act on the serotonin system and have very little anticholinergic activity. Since the majority of serotonin is located in the gastrointestinal tract, serotonergic medication can be a cause of abdominal pain, nausea, diarrhea, and flatulence. Gastrointestinal disturbances are usually transient, and they can be minimized by using lower doses or delayed-release preparations.

Sexual Dysfunction

Sexual dysfunction caused by SSRIs consists of decreased libido, inability to orgasm, and impaired ejaculation and erection. Even though sexual dysfunction is amongst the more common side effects, patients often do not report it spontaneously. Therefore, it is important to ask the patient specifically about this side effect. Some patients find this side effect unacceptable. In such cases, it can be beneficial for the treatment plan to switch to another medication that is not associated with sexual dysfunction.

Weight Gain

Psychotropic drugs cause retention of fluid, increase of caloric intake, alteration of metabolism, and a decrease in the amount of exercise. These factors are associated with an increase in weight, which is a common reason for treatment non-compliance. In certain cases, weight gain can be a sign of recovery (e.g., bulimia nervosa). Olanzapine and valproate cause insulin resistance, which increases appetite, and therefore increases weight. Metformin can make weight loss possible in patients who gain weight as a consequence of treatment with serotonin-dopamine reuptake inhibitors and valproic acid. SSRIs can cause weight loss at the beginning of treatment. However, the weight is usually regained in the first few months.

Chapter 17: Psychoeducational Group Facilitation

Psychoeducational Groups

Psychoeducational groups can be defined as groups that focus on the education of a wide range of audiences on a psychological concept or topic. These groups can be used with children, adolescents, and adults. They can be practiced in various types of settings such as hospitals, universities, social service agencies, etc. The leader of a psychoeducational group should have a firm grasp on a wide variety of knowledge, expertise, and skills needed to guide a diverse audience. The leaders of psychoeducational groups should provide guidance for personal learning, show members how to decrease isolation and help each other, foster hope, promote self-awareness, find opportunities for new learning, and create a safe space for emotional expression.

KASST Model

The KASST Model consists of several categories that include knowledge, art, science, skills, and techniques. In the facilitation of a psychoeducational group, these categories are not isolated but blended. Every category provides important guidance in your development as a group leader. Mastery of these categories will make you a competent group leader.

Since psychoeducational groups deal with various audiences, group leaders should have a firm knowledge base concerning groups, topics, or conditions that the group focuses on. This is necessary to be able to teach the group. Just like every group member is an entity, the group as a whole should also be considered as an entity. The group leader should understand the wholeness of the group. Group leaders need to have knowledge about the group dynamics, stages of development, therapeutic factors, processes, ethics, instructional principles, and conditions or topics.

The art of the group depends on the group leader's self-awareness and personal development. The authentic self of the group leader manifests through their expression of warmth, tolerance, respect, caring, and genuineness. Group members can sense the authenticity of the group leader. Your personal development impacts many aspects such as cultural sensitivity, countertransference, and unconscious negative impact. Group leaders are encouraged to be introspective and work on potentially unresolved issues.

The science component refers to the framework and support of the group, which includes activities that will assist as you plan, organize, structure, direct, and evaluate. The instructional part is necessary to achieve optimal function and group facilitation.

The group leader should be competent in basic interview, communication, and counseling skills. However, skills are not a replacement for knowledge, understanding, and self-development of the group leader.

Techniques are strategies that help you in teaching and group facilitation. Some techniques include activities like games, role-play, and exercises or teaching approaches like discussions and media. Other examples of techniques are the facilitation of procedures like conflict resolution. Techniques can promote learning, retention, and participant involvement. Techniques should be used thoughtfully, and not as a replacement for reflection and deeper understanding of personal issues and relationships. Using activities only to reduce the anxiety of the group leader is counterproductive.

Group Leader Self-Factors, Competencies, and Skills

The art factors of group leadership cannot be learned since they depend on the individual development of the group leader. Personal development has a direct and indirect impact on your clients. It can prevent burnout and countertransference, facilitate a better understanding of client's issues, and promote confidence in dealing with issues. Unresolved issues stem from childhood experiences and past life events that influence the ways you react to and manage criticism, your perceptions about yourself and others, and your beliefs, attitudes, and values. Developing self-awareness is important because the more you understand yourself, the more you will understand your clients.

Transference and Countertransference

Transference and countertransference are defined as processes through which one's thoughts, feelings, and wishes are transferred onto another person. Transference occurs when the process is transferred from a group member to the group leader. Countertransference occurs when the process is transferred from the group leader to the group member. These processes are unconscious, and therefore they can be hard to identify.

Countertransference can be detrimental to the relationship with group members. Countertransference impacts the group leader's perception of the client, their reaction, the direction of sessions, and objectivity. An example of countertransference will be shown to clarify this process. Imagine you and your father had a close relationship, but they died in an accident when you were only ten years old. Throughout the years you have managed to process some of your grief, but you are still influenced by that loss and you wish you had your father with you. A group member who is much younger than you expresses that they hate their father because he is emotionally and verbally abusive. Hearing this, you start to feel angry but you attempt to suppress it. You respond calmly and you say that their father is probably trying to help them build a more meaningful life, and they should be more appreciative and understanding of how hard it is to be a parent. This response makes the group members feel misunderstood, and they withdraw. Countertransference can be prevented by bringing unresolved unconscious issues to conscious awareness and processing them.

Underdeveloped Narcissism or Self-Absorption

Unhealthy narcissism stems from an overdevelopment of self-importance and a lack of proper self-regulation. Narcissism is characterized by a lack of empathy and disrespect for other's boundaries. Narcissistic behavior impacts the ability to understand others and get in touch with what they are experiencing. This can have a detrimental effect on the group dynamics. Examples of narcissistic behavior include interrupting someone in the middle of a conversation or using someone's possessions without asking them first.

Basic Leader Characteristics

Group members may have trust issues. They may wonder if participating in a psychoeducational group will benefit them. The group leader should have a deep belief in the group process. This will unconsciously provide reassurance and relief to the group members. The group leader should have confidence in their group leadership abilities. They should be able to take risks and expose themselves to potential failures. The group leader should accept criticism from others and always be ready for change and growth. The group leader should be willing to admit mistakes and imperfections. This ability conveys to group members a model of self-acceptance and self-compassion. The group leader should effectively plan and organize. They should be flexible and able to tolerate anxiety. Inflexible leaders can make the group members feel controlled. As mentioned earlier, group leaders should be able to introspect and develop self-awareness. Personal ownership means the ability to take responsibility for yourself and your behaviors, feelings, opinions, and attitudes. The group leader should also have a sense of humor since laughing can relieve tension and promote a sense of playfulness. Basic inner self characteristics are part of one's integral self and include caring, warmth, positive regard, and genuineness. They are manifested through nonverbal behaviors such as maintained eye contact, appropriate facial expressions, smiles, etc.

Group Leadership Skills

Attending skills are conveyed through nonverbal behaviors such as eye contact, orientation of your body toward the speaker, and leaning forward. This shows members that you are interested in what they have to say. Group leaders should develop active listening and response skills, and the ability to reflect, clarify, and summarize the key elements of the session. The group leader should learn when to provide support and when to leave members to work through issues on their own.

The Group: Process and Progress

Group leaders should understand the group as a whole and be able to respond in a timely manner as the session unfolds. When key events during sessions are missed, this can harm the group and make group members feel ignored. This can be prevented by learning about group dynamics, group stages, and helpful group factors. These components do not occur in isolation, and they can change from moment to moment.

Group Dynamics

Group dynamics is the process of the group that includes the level of participation, resistance, relationship between members and between members and the leader, communication patterns, nonverbal behaviors, and feelings expressed.

The cooperation and interaction between members and the leader, the contribution of members, and the member's level of functioning determines the level of participation. Do members participate? Do they look reluctant and withdrawn or are they active? When does their involvement change? Do some members become energized after a discussion? Do some members become silent after a discussion? The group leader should observe the group dynamics since they can help determine the needs of the group members.

Resistance is a normal occurrence during the group process. When a group member shows resistance, you should move on to another topic or person. If the whole group is resistant, you can explore this by starting a discussion about the usefulness of the activity. You should not try to break down the resistance.

In the beginning, it is expected that group members will communicate through the leader. You can encourage communication between members by asking them to talk to each other directly. Some members may feel excluded from the communication. You can include them by asking for their input. Group members can communicate in a warm, supportive way or in a cold and hostile way. Some members appear aloof or tentative when they communicate. You should observe individual communication patterns as well as group patterns.

Members will expect the group leader to provide for their needs and expectations. Some members seek the leader's approval. Facilitation of relationships between group members can be achieved by empowering members to take charge of their learning.

Nonverbal signals, or metacommunication, are thought to be a more accurate representation of an individual's internal state than verbal communication. Nonverbal communication includes postures, gestures, eye contact, voice tones, and others.

The feeling tone of the group can give you an idea of how group members are progressing. To determine the feeling tone, the group leader should develop self-awareness, which requires being attuned to your feelings as a possible reflection of what the others are feeling.

Problem Behaviors

Problem behaviors in psychoeducational groups can be divided into overparticipation, underparticipation, socializing, and disengagement.

Members who overparticipate will often interrupt other members while they are speaking, engage in distracting behaviors, and monopolize the attention of the group leader. At the start of the process, it may be useful to have a member who overparticipates since they may engage and energize the other group members. However, their over-involvement usually becomes a problem. The group leader should find a way to reduce overparticipating behavior without offending the overparticipating member.

Members who underparticipate are withdrawn, silent, and often make very few responses even when you ask them a direct question. Underparticipating members usually do the minimum required when participating in activities. Underparticipation occurs as a self-protection or rebellion response. These members often did not choose to be in the group (e.g., court-ordered participants), and therefore, they refused to participate in it. The group leader should not force them, and they should acknowledge that you cannot force all members to participate. You can offer them opportunities that will give them the chance to involve themselves in the group, but you cannot push them.

The socializing members tend to engage in conversations while other members are talking, they frequently interact with the same people. They can introduce different topics while something else is being discussed. Rather than participate in activities, they tend to start conversations and are frequently late when coming back from breaks. A group usually has two or more socializers. In counseling/therapy groups, often the other group members may confront the socializers. You can deal with socializers by physically being near them, talking to them about their behavior, or making sure they are placed in different groups.

Disengaged members can disengage themselves from the group physically, mentally, or emotionally. Examples of physical disengagement include absence, being late, leaning back into the chair, or premature termination. An example of mental disengagement is daydreaming. Examples of emotional disengagement include changing the topic, not maintaining eye contact, asking rhetorical questions, intellectualizing, or becoming numb. Due to the short-term nature of psychoeducational groups, it may be hard to effectively manage disengaging behaviors.

Chapter 18: Health Promotion

Promotion of mental health can help people manage life situations and events more easily, regardless of whether they are predictable or unpredictable. Mental health promotion can help patients increase their self-esteem and well-being. Health promotion involves work with individuals, groups, and communities. The psychiatric mental health nurse practitioner teaches people to improve their life skills as well as their quality of life. The psychiatric mental health nurse practitioner should also aim to influence social, economic, and environmental factors that influence mental health. The promotion of mental health aims to develop positive mental health for individuals with mental health problems and the community in general. An individual's mental health is tied to their relationship with other people, their lifestyle, the degree of power they have over their lives, and environmental factors.

Models of Health Promotion

According to Tannahill, there are three models of health promotion. The first model is based on the radical humanist and structuralist theoretical approach. The second approach is based on health persuasion, community development, personal counseling, and legislative action. The third model is based on disease management, disease prevention, politics of health (social action, economic management, and policy), and health education. The five strategies for health promotion include medical, behavioral change, empowerment, educational, and social change.

Mental health promotion is done on both an individual and population level. Promoting the mental health of populations can be done through various interventions such as prevention, treatment, maintenance, and continuing care.

Goals of Health Promotion

Mental health promotion is focused on the promotion of the emotional and social well-being of people without mental illness, people who are at risk of mental illness, and people who are experiencing mental illness. Goals of health promotion include protection, support, and sustainability of social and emotional well-being, promotion of mentally healthy lifestyles, and support of productive and meaningful lives. Health promotion aims to increase people's sense of belonging and connectedness. It builds resilience by increasing protective factors and reducing risk factors that can be threatening to emotional and social well-being. Health promotion improves coping skills and adaptations of individuals and communities, especially in the face of adversity. Health promotion enables healthy communities, workplaces, schools, and social supports and builds community acceptance and tolerance by increasing the understanding of cultural, personal, social, and spiritual differences.

Mental Health Prevention

Mental health prevention can be defined as interventions that are done before the onset of a mental illness, that aim to prevent its development. These interventions can target specific life stages in order to reduce the development of mental illness during life cycle transitions and age-associated onset. Prevention can target the individual or populations. It can be divided into primary, secondary, and tertiary prevention. The main goals of mental health prevention are to reduce the incidence and prevalence of certain psychiatric disorders (primary and secondary prevention), to reduce or delay the recurrence, frequency, and interval of psychiatric disorders (relapse prevention), and to reduce the time a patient spends with a psychiatric disorder, the impact and severity of the disorder, and the distress, pain, and suffering associated with the psychiatric disorder (treatment, recovery, secondary, and tertiary prevention).

Mental health prevention can reduce risk factors, social and environmental conditions, and high-risk behaviors that are associated with psychiatric disorders.

Relapse Prevention

Relapse prevention helps people to stay in a good state after a first or subsequent episode of a psychiatric disorder. Relapse prevention aims to prevent or reduce the recurrence of a disorder and the exacerbation of symptoms. Relapse prevention does not only include medication adherence and psychoeducation, but also promotion of awareness, resilience, and recovery. What happens to the patient while they are in remission can have a big impact on prevention. This includes life experiences, development and growth, risk factors, protective factors, the environment, and social circumstances.

The successful relapse prevention plan consists of a few components. In order to achieve relapse prevention, the healthcare staff should increase awareness – recognize and accept the illness, and motivate the patient to change. The relapse signature should be identified, which means that the staff should recognize triggers and warning signs of the occurrence of an episode or crisis. Responsibilities should be divided and mutual collaboration should be encouraged. You should work with the patient to identify personal preferences and future options. The types of behaviors that should be continued or avoided is an important factor in the achievement of a state of healthy maintenance. Early intervention is an important component that consists of self-action, re-engaging, stabilization, and access to services. Patients should be empowered and the staff should help them build resilience during remission.

Building Resilience

Patients differ in their ability to cope with adverse situations and avoid breaking down when confronted with stressful events. Responses to stress are often coping mechanisms. Coping and defensive mechanisms can be healthy or maladaptive. Resilience is an interactive dynamic process that emerges as a product of the environment the person is living in and their constitution. Protective factors help people cope with stressors and enable them to modify their behaviors. Protective factors are not always visible and may only become detectable when the person is faced with a stressor.

Identifying risk factors for mental illness is an important component in the development of resilience. Risk factors should be identified early in the psychosocial and mental health assessment. They can help the clinician determine risk management, scope of intervention, and care planning. Identification of risk factors can help strengthen resilience at both the individual and community level. Risk factor prevention can be incorporated into prevention programs, targeted mental health literacy and educational programs, screening for at-risk groups, and social interventions.

Common risk factors include poor or interrupted development or maturity, unstable and dysfunctional interpersonal relationships, absent or poor parenting, family discord, domestic violence and abuse, parent(s) with severe psychiatric disorder and disability, overwhelming adversity or grief and loss, loneliness, lack of peer and social support, lack of friends, drug or alcohol use, poor nutrition, poor sleep, social exclusion, social disadvantage, injustice, poverty, stigma, and persistent physical disability.

Incorporating the development of protective factors when caring for patients can help them achieve a higher level of functioning, prevent the recurrence of their illness, decrease psychiatric disability and social isolation, develop coping skills, and promote optimum recovery. At the community level, resilience and protective factors can be promoted through anti-bullying programs in schools, healthy working environments, promotion of healthy lifestyles, self-help, and personal growth, development courses, mental health literacy, teaching people about emotional intelligence, and connecting people in the community with ethnic minorities and the socially disadvantaged. By building resilience at the community level, you can increase emotional well-being in society.

Common protective factors include a healthy lifestyle, nurturing and affectionate family relationships, positive school and work environments, social "connectedness" and belonging, reliable friendships and social support networks, a positive "temperament" (humor, patience, hope, and tolerance), emotional intelligence, self-awareness, self-esteem, acceptance, opportunities and achievements, and the presence of mentors or personal encouragements.

Teaching resilience, reducing risk factors, and strengthening protective factors will enable patients to cope with unexpected adverse events, and increase their ability to adapt to life circumstances. Teaching resilience, reducing risk factors, and strengthening protective factors will enable patients to cope with unexpected adverse events and increase their ability to adapt to life circumstances. Resilience enables people to accept and understand themselves, understand their illness and learn to live with it, take responsibility for their health, and develop adaptability to stress.

Interventions

Tobacco Cessation

The mental health nurse should assess the negative impact of smoking on the patient's health and intervene to reduce that impact. Tobacco smoking is associated with many health issues and a shorter life expectancy. The management of tobacco use is done through cessation programs, prevention of exposure to second-hand smoke, prevention of smoking in young populations, and changing the population's attitudes toward smoking.

Nicotine is among the most addictive substances, and therefore it can be extremely difficult to quit. Quitting nicotine may require multiple attempts and different cessation methods. There are nicotine-based medications that are used as nicotine-replacement therapy. These include nicotine gums, patches, inhalers, and lozenges. Varenicline and bupropion are non-nicotine-based medications that can be helpful for long-term cessation. Counseling combined with medication is more effective than counseling or medication alone.

You should assess for tobacco use in patients who are admitted to the hospital. During hospitalization, patients who are addicted to nicotine will experience withdrawal symptoms if they do not have access to nicotine-replacement products. Therefore, they should be provided nicotine replacement therapy, such as nicotine gums or patches.

Nurses should discuss tobacco use with every patient. Assessment of tobacco use should be done at every admission. You should ask every smoker whether they have an intention to quit smoking. If they do, refer them to services that help with cessation. Encourage the use of apps and quitlines and offer health education to every tobacco user. Every patient should have an individualized quitting plan. The quitting plan should include both short-term and long-term goals for quitting and strategies to avoid exposure to secondhand smoke.

Self-Care

Mental health is not defined only by the absence of illness but by the presence of emotional, psychological, and social well-being. Self-care is one of the ways people can maintain their mental health and prevent the onset of a psychiatric illness. Self-care can help patients with an existing mental illness to support their treatment goals and recovery. There are many self-care recommendations that you can present to patients.

You should advise patients to get regular exercise, at least thirty minutes per day. Regular exercise is known to improve mood, mental health, and cognitive abilities. Patients should be advised to eat healthy and balanced meals with regular hydration. This will improve their focus and increase their energy throughout the day. They should also limit caffeinated beverages and beverages with high sugar content.

You should educate patients about the importance of sleep. Patients should be advised to stick to a regular sleeping schedule and minimize exposure to blue light before bedtime since that can affect their circadian rhythm. You should educate patients about relaxation techniques and introduce them to wellness programs or apps, which teach patients how to meditate and practice progressive muscle relaxation, or breathing exercises. Patients should be educated on the importance of other self-care activities such as journaling.

By setting realistic goals and priorities, patients can make a balanced use of their time. They should be taught to say "no" when new tasks start piling up, since taking on too much can easily cause burnout. Another method that can be beneficial for a person's mental health is practicing gratitude and keeping a gratitude journal. Patients should remind themselves daily of things for which they are grateful. This will foster positive emotions. Teach patients to focus on the positive things in their lives and teach them to identify negative thoughts that may be affecting their mood. Connection is another major factor that influences mental health. Remind patients to reach out to family and friends when they need emotional support or help.

Every patient is different in their self-care needs and preferences. You should explain to patients that they need to find what they genuinely enjoy and that what works for one person may not work for another. Self-care does not cure mental illness, but it can help people cope and manage their mental health better.

Patients need to know when to seek professional help. Inform patients that they should seek professional help if they have been experiencing severe symptoms for two weeks or more. Distressing and severe symptoms include difficulty sleeping, changes in appetite that have resulted in weight gain or loss, struggle to get out of bed due to mood changes, issues with concentration and focus, issues with daily functioning, and a loss of interest in previously enjoyable activities.

Chapter 19: Emergent Situations and Crisis Management

Psychiatric emergencies require immediate therapeutic intervention. The incidence of emergency psychiatry patients is increasing due to various reasons such as the rising prevalence of mental health disorders, substance use disorders, and socioeconomic factors like homelessness and unemployment. Emergency psychiatry deals with issues such as violence (homicide, suicide, and rape), substance abuse, abuse of children and spouses, and social issues (competence, homelessness, and aging). The most common diagnoses seen in the psychiatric emergency department are mood disorders (depression and manic episodes), schizophrenia, and alcohol dependence. This chapter will provide a general overview of psychiatric emergencies as well as crisis management.

Treatment Settings

The setting in which the emergency psychiatric evaluation is done must have an atmosphere of safety and security. The staff consists of psychiatrists, nurses, aides, and social workers. The staff should be present at all times. There should be additional personnel that will help out in cases of overcrowding. The emergency team should be educated and trained on the proper practice of restraints.

One-third of medical conditions may present with psychiatric manifestations. Therefore, the staff should have access to the medical emergency department. Psychopharmacological treatment options must be available to the prescribing clinician.

Patients who present with physical or emotional distress are in a vulnerable position. Their fantasies or unrealistic expectations can influence their response to treatment. For example, a person who is in psychosis may not understand that the healthcare staff is there to help him. Therefore, all actions taken by the healthcare staff should have this in consideration and try to minimize the potential for misunderstandings.

Evaluation

The emergency psychiatry evaluation consists of the standard psychiatric interview (history and mental status examination), a full physical examination, and additional tests (as needed). However, certain modifications in the evaluation may be necessary. For example, if the clinician is evaluating a rambling manic patient, they may need to alter the structure of the interview. An agitated patient may have to be restrained. When assessing a patient's risk of suicide, the usual rules of confidentiality may need to be abandoned. The reason behind the modification should be documented in the medical record.

The clinicians can protect themselves by knowing about the patients as much as possible before the meeting, by being on high alert for potential violence, having others present in their vicinity, and developing an alliance with the patient (e.g., do not threaten a patient with persecutory delusions). It is also important to be safe in the physical environment (e.g., by having open access to the door).

The staff should aim to prevent any type of harm. Use the least restrictive methods necessary to prevent the patient from injuring themselves, which may include physical restraint as a last resort. Violence toward others must also be prevented. First, the patient's risk of violence should be assessed. If there is a risk of violence, the patient should first be reassured and calmed in a non-threatening way. Medication should be offered if verbal de-escalation fails. When both pharmacotherapy and verbal de-escalation fail, the staff may be required to use physical restraints. If there is a need to use restraints, you should inform the patient beforehand. When the patient is restrained, regularly observe them and check their vital signs. Restrained patients should be isolated from agitating stimuli.

Medical or Psychiatric?

Emergency situations can have a medical, psychiatric, or both medical and psychiatric etiology. Medical conditions that cause mental status changes that resemble mental illness include diabetes mellitus, acute intoxications, withdrawal, thyroid disease, AIDS, and head traumas. Medical conditions can be life-threatening and they generally have a more definitive treatment with a better prognosis. Some factors that point toward a medical cause of a psychiatric presentation include acute onset, older age at onset, the first episode, the presence of a comorbid medical illness or injury, nonauditory hallucinations, mental status signs (e.g., disorientation, reduced alertness, impairment of memory, concentration, and attention, speech problems), history of significant substance abuse, neurologic symptoms (e.g., loss of consciousness, change in vision, head injury, seizures), and constructional apraxia (e.g., the patient is struggling to draw a clock).

Specific Situations

The Violent Patient

Violence can be caused by various reasons. The underlying reason behind violent behavior has implications for the choice of interventions. The differential diagnosis of violent behavior is wide and includes medical causes (cerebral neoplasms, infections, temporal lobe epilepsy), personality disorders (antisocial personality disorders, paranoid personality disorder, decompensating obsessive-compulsive personality disorder), dissociative disorders, delusional disorder, bipolar disorder, violence due to interpersonal stress, schizophrenia, psychoactive substance-induced organic mental disorder, alcohol intoxication, and others. Certain signs that might alert the clinician of impending violence include recent acts of violence, history of violent behavior, threats (verbal or physical), progressive psychomotor agitation, alcohol or drug intoxication, persecutory ideation in a psychotic patient, catatonic excitement, history of violent acts, and a history of childhood abuse.

During the interview, the clinician should make a differential diagnosis of violent behavior and attempt to predict the risk of violence. You should consider violent ideation - does the patient have a wish, plan, intent, and available means such as weapons? The demographic is also an important factor since violent patients are most often young male patients with low socioeconomic status and few social supports. Patients with a history of violence, nonviolent antisocial acts, and low impulse control have an increased risk of violence. The presence of interpersonal stressors in the patient's life (e.g., marital conflict) is another important predictor.

Violence can come from aggression or agitation. Aggression is organized and purposeful, and it often results because of conflict. Aggression is less likely to be because of a mental disorder. The psychiatric interview can be used as a screening tool to determine whether threats of violence have a psychiatric origin. Aggressive patients may require legal intervention.

Agitation can be defined as a state of tension or restlessness that can result in purposeless and disorganized violent behavior. Agitation is usually associated with an underlying medical or psychiatric condition. Confusion and fear cause a state of agitation. De-escalation is the primary goal in dealing with an agitated patient. Verbal de-escalation is attempted at first. Simple sentences are helpful since they are more likely to be understood by confused patients. Pharmacologic medication with benzodiazepines or antipsychotics can be used when verbal de-escalation fails. If both measures fail, the staff may be required to use physical restraints. Restraints should be used only in extreme circumstances since they cause both physical and psychological trauma.

The Depressed and Potentially Suicidal Patient

Suicide is the leading cause of death in teenagers and young adults. All psychiatric disorders increase the risk of suicide. During the mental state examination, the clinician should directly ask every patient who presents with a mental health concern if they have suicidal thoughts or ideas. The majority of patients who have intent to commit suicide give a warning about their plan. Therefore, direct questions (e.g., Are you suicidal?) should be asked regularly to assess suicidality risk. Signs that indicate an increased risk of suicide include a history of suicidal attempt(s), a history of suicidal ideation, availability of means of suicide, a family history, pervasive pessimism or hopelessness, a concern for the effect of suicide on family members, verbalized suicidal ideation, life crisis, preparation of a will, admitting to a plan of action, and resignation after agitated depression (e.g., a patient who was previously threatening suicide suddenly becomes quiet).

As with any patient who presents with a psychiatric emergency, ensuring safety is a priority. Patients who have an imminent risk of suicidal behavior must be hospitalized or protected in another way. Involuntary hospitalization may be needed in patients who are a danger to themselves. In certain patients, the risk is not immediate but there is potential for suicide if the patient continues to be depressed. In these situations, if the patient is not hospitalized, the clinician should insist that the patient contacts their healthcare team if suicidal ideation increases. Hospitalized patients may need intensive monitoring and observation which may include the presence of a one-to-one "sitter." In the inpatient setting, you must make sure that the patient does not have access to any means by which they can harm themselves such as glass or other sharp items. A physical examination should be done to search for signs of self-injurious behavior (e.g., if the patient has cut themselves or has jumped off a building). Patients who come to the hospital with suicidal ideation may have already attempted it by ingesting substances in order to overdose. Since the effects of overdose are not apparent in the first hours after ingestion, you should order labs (e.g., acetylsalicylic acid level) to assess for an occult overdose. Remember that patients with suicidal ideation can also have medical problems. Therefore, consider that they may need medical hospitalization.

Not all patients who present with suicidal ideation need hospitalization. The determination of who is safe to go home and who should be hospitalized is a challenge for all psychiatric healthcare staff. If there is a chance that the patient may attempt suicide shortly, they require 24/7 monitoring and treatment. Hospitalization can treat the underlying mental illness that is contributing to the risk of suicide. Factors that increase the likelihood of a suicide attempt shortly include access to guns, use of ethanol or other substances that increase impulsivity, recent suicide attempt(s), ongoing thoughts of suicide, and recent self-harm.

Rape and Sexual Abuse

Rape and sexual abuse can cause consequences that might last a lifetime. Rape is often a life-threatening experience since victims are almost always threatened with physical harm. A weapon is often involved. Rape includes sexual intercourse, anal intercourse, and oral sex. The majority of rapists are male, while the majority of victims are female. In institutions such as prisons, male rape also occurs. The category most at risk of rape is females between the ages of sixteen and twenty-four.

The normal reactions of rape victims include humiliation, shame, anxiety, confusion, and outrage. Many victims feel partially responsible for the assault. The clinician who evaluates a rape and sexual abuse victim should provide reassurance and support in a nonjudgmental way. If possible, when the victim is female, the clinician should be female since victims may feel uncomfortable speaking to a man. The clinician should inform the victim about medical and legal services, as well as rape crisis centers that can provide multidisciplinary services, including counseling and support groups. The clinician should be aware that the victim has undergone life-threatening stress. The evaluation requires meticulous documentation since the medical record can be used as evidence during prosecutions.

Pharmacotherapy

Indications for pharmacotherapy in psychiatric emergencies include violence or assault, panic or massive anxiety, and extrapyramidal reactions (e.g., dystonia, akathisia). Tranquilization is needed for delusional patients and patients who are in a state of catatonic excitement. Antipsychotics, benzodiazepines, and antihistamines can be used for episodic outbursts of violence. Intoxication from drugs of abuse can be treated with conservative measures. Haloperidol is given five to ten mg every half-hour to an hour in certain patients who need to be stabilized. If the drug that caused the intoxication has anticholinergic properties, it is better to use benzodiazepines instead of antipsychotics.

For violent patients, you may give five to ten mg diazepam or two to four mg lorazepam, intravenously over two minutes. When administering IV medication, the nurse should take great care to avoid causing respiratory arrest. Haloperidol (five to ten mg) can be given intramuscularly for patients who require IM medication. Continuous medication is indicated in cases where the symptoms come back after the IV medication wears off. Using large doses initially results in an overmedicated patient. Therefore, giving small IM or oral doses at half-hour to one-hour intervals is more appropriate. The patient's vital signs should be monitored at all times during treatment.

Chapter 20: Intervention Effectiveness

General Considerations in Intervention Selection

Healthcare providers should be aware of general considerations that play an important role in treatment selection, regardless of the circumstances in which the patient is presenting.

Treatment Effectiveness

Most psychotherapy treatments are effective. However, some are more effective than others. For example, highly focused treatments (e.g., systematic desensitization for the treatment of phobias) are more effective than treatments with a wide focus (e.g., client-centered care in the development of personal growth goals). Factors that influence treatment effectiveness include the specific therapy techniques, the patient's expectations of the outcome, the patient's characteristics, the patient's circumstances and environment, and others.

Clinical Expertise

The clinical expertise of the clinician who is treating the patient consists of his/her diagnostic competence, clinical decision-making, case formulation, treatment planning and implementation, monitoring of progress, interpersonal skills, incorporation of new knowledge and skills, and continuous self-reflection. A clinician with a high clinical expertise has a higher chance of achieving a good outcome.

Cultural Considerations

The patient's culture needs to be taken into consideration when prescribing and beginning treatment. Certain guidelines can help clinicians practice cultural adaptation in the treatment process. The services that clinicians provide should be meaningful in the cultural context in which they are being delivered. Before implementing treatment, clinicians should conduct cultural assessments. They should use traditional treatments as existing resources and communicate in a culturally appropriate empathetic manner. Cultural differences are not deficits and should not be interpreted as such.

Patient Preferences

The majority of patients want to actively participate in the treatment plan development. They want to be able to actively make decisions. Clinicians should be aware of patients' preferences. Patients can have three types of preferences: role, therapist, and treatment-type preferences. Role preferences refer to the expectations that patients have from the clinician's behavior. Some patients prefer that the therapist provides a listening role, while others prefer a more active advice-giving role. Therapist preferences refer to the preferences related to the clinician's characteristics. For example, some patients prefer that the therapist comes from a similar ethnic background. Some patients prefer therapists who have many years of clinical experience, while others prefer younger therapists. Treatment-type preferences refer to the preferences about the specific type of intervention that the patient expects to receive. Some patients prefer a behavioral approach, while others prefer a cognitive approach. Some patients prefer a pharmacological approach, while some expect the best results from a psychotherapeutic approach. Patient preferences play a major role in the treatment outcome.

Patient Expectations

The expectations for the treatment outcome are another important aspect of treatment planning. It is normal for patients to arrive at treatment with certain expectations. Patients have expectations of what will be required of them, what the likely outcome will be, how much time it will take to achieve that outcome, the clinician's responsibilities, the relationship between the clinician and the patient, and other factors. Factors that influence patient expectations include the patient's personality, previous experiences with mental health treatment, whether treatment is voluntary or involuntary, and what kind of information they have obtained through the media or others.

Being aware of the patient's expectations can have a positive impact on the patient-provider relationship. The clinician should also communicate their expectations for the type of treatment to the patient. By communicating both the patient's and the clinician's expectations for the treatment options, both patient and clinician can develop a plan that is realistic, achievable, and acceptable.

Comorbid Medical/Psychiatric Disorders

Patients who have one or more comorbid medical or psychiatric disorders, can be challenging to treat. Clinicians frequently treat patients who have maladaptive ways of thinking, coping, or behaving, and patients with personality disorders or cognitive impairment due to neurologic disease. Comorbid disorders can become significant barriers to an effective intervention plan.

Clinicians should pay special attention during the development of the treatment plan to comorbid medical disorders that are often accompanied by anxiety, depression, or other psychiatric symptoms (e.g., asthma, diabetes, congestive heart failure). The clinician should make an effort to have close coordination with the patient's medical care team. The clinician should consider the physical and psychological symptoms of the disorder that may interfere with the treatment they plan to prescribe. For example, patients who have suffered a stroke may be limited in mobility due to paralysis, and this may impair their ability to use behavioral techniques. If the stroke has resulted in speech deficits, these patients may have difficulties with therapeutic techniques that involve verbal expression. Patients with a condition that limits physical endurance (e.g., severe emphysema) may benefit from briefer but more frequent sessions.

Healthcare providers (physicians, clinical nurse practitioners, physician assistants) in nonpsychiatric medical professions have become more sensitive to psychiatric issues in their patients. Because of this, the number of referrals to psychiatry has increased. This means that healthcare providers are seeing more patients with comorbid medical conditions. Therefore, psychiatric healthcare providers should be educated on the common physical diseases and disorders, and consider them in the treatment plan development.

Specific Intervention Decisions

The clinician needs to be aware of several treatment aspects in order to choose the best appropriate intervention for the patient he/she is treating. The most appropriate intervention will result in the achievement of the mutually agreed-upon goals and objectives.

Appropriate Level of Care (LOC)

An appropriate level of care according to the patient's circumstances is the first consideration when planning a specific treatment for a patient. Factors that influence the LOC are the severity of the patient's problems, the effectiveness of the treatment and intensity level appropriate for the problem, and the treatment's availability. The patient can receive treatment at several LOCs which include residential, partial hospitalization, 23-hour bed, intensive outpatient, and outpatient care.

Specific tools that help clinicians decide the appropriate LOC can be used. For example, the American Society of Addiction Medicine's (ASAM) Criteria helps healthcare providers determine the LOC for patients with psychiatric and substance use disorders. The LOCAT can assist in determining the severity of symptoms and conditions, whether there is acute danger present, psychosocial factors, mental status changes, functional impairment, and additional factors (e.g., history of violence, response to treatment). Choosing the inappropriate LOC can cause stagnation or worsening of the patient's condition.

Type/Mode of Intervention

Psychotherapeutic

"Talk therapy" is first-line treatment for patients who seek help for substance abuse or mental health issues. Psychotherapeutic formats include individual therapy, group therapy, family therapy, etc. Some patients benefit the most from individual therapy. Some patients may see the best results from group therapy.

The optimal type of psychotherapy depends on several factors. For example, a couple who is seeking help for their marital problems will benefit the most from conjoint marital therapy. A patient who has problems connecting and relating to others will see the most benefits from group therapy. For some patients, the best approach would be a combination of modalities (e.g., individual and family therapy), while for some the preferred approach is a succession of modalities (e.g., seven sessions of individual psychotherapy followed by ten sessions of family therapy).

In certain cases, the appropriate LOC will dictate the type of therapeutic intervention. For example, a patient who is hospitalized because of a suicide attempt may benefit from individual and group therapy. However, that may be impractical during an inpatient stay.

Psychopharmacologic

Many patients present with symptoms that cannot be alleviated without psychopharmacologic interventions. Medications are the most effective treatments for some disorders, either alone or in combination with another therapeutic modality. Psychopharmacologic intervention is a good approach for patients who suffer from major depressive disorder, attention-deficit/hyperactivity disorder, or psychotic disorders.

The decision whether to use medication or not depends on several factors. These include the patient's motivation and ability to follow a psychopharmacologic treatment regimen, whether the patient's condition can be treated without medication, whether the medication is effective for the specific symptoms, financial burden, tolerability of side effects, and the presence of other conditions (medical or psychiatric) that contraindicate the use of medications. The clinician should weigh the potential costs and benefits when implementing a psychopharmacologic intervention.

Medical

Other than psychopharmacologic treatment, the patient may require other types of pharmacologic treatment or other medical interventions. Sometimes, the patient may need to be referred to another medical specialty. Certain patients may benefit from procedures such as electroconvulsive therapy (ECT) or neurosurgeries (e.g., deep brain stimulation).

The psychiatrist should be aware that the patient's treatment goals can be made easier to achieve through other medical interventions for physical conditions (e.g., control of hyperglycemia with insulin). The psychiatrist should be sensitive to the presence of comorbid medical conditions and refer the patient when needed.

Educational

The psychiatrist can offer the patient many educational resources as adjuncts to the therapeutic intervention. Examples include interactive websites, college courses, workshops, books, and other resources that can help the patient educate themself about their condition and ways to manage it. A knowledgeable patient may be more collaborative, and this will make the treatment process more effective.

Other Modes of Intervention

Some patients may benefit from additional modes of intervention. Examples include community self-help and support groups, retreats focused on specific topics, between-session homework assignments, telepsychology websites, and others. Incorporation of these activities may be beneficial for the treatment process. However, they should not be treated as the primary treatment modality for any patient.

Multimodal/Eclectic/Integrative approach

The most commonly implemented multimodal approach is the combination of psychopharmacologic and psychotherapeutic interventions. Clinicians can combine various types of psychotherapy. Patients with marital problems are frequently treated by combining individual psychotherapy and marital therapy. Patients with problems in interpersonal relationships are frequently treated with a combination of individual and group therapy.

The clinician can prescribe different approaches to one type of treatment. For example, different individual psychotherapeutic approaches can be incorporated into the treatment of one patient. A patient who suffers from a specific phobia can be treated by combining behavioral therapy (e.g., implosion or desensitization) and cognitive therapy (e.g., rational emotive therapy). For this patient, behavior therapy can help alleviate distressing symptoms while cognitive therapy can help restructure maladaptive cognitive beliefs. Sometimes, it is appropriate to use one type of therapeutic approach in the initial phases of treatment and another approach in the later stage of treatment.

Determination of which treatment approach is the most appropriate depends on many factors. The clinician should be flexible and open to considering the various treatment approaches that can effectively result in a good outcome for the patient.

Evidence-Based Approaches to Treatment

Choosing the most effective and appropriate treatment for every individual patient is a challenging task. Clinicians have access to empirically based guides to treatment for most of the problems they encounter in clinical practice.

Clinical Practice Guidelines

Clinical practice guidelines are systematically developed declarations that support certain treatment actions or approaches. Guidelines are a representation of a consensus of experts who have agreed upon what the best treatment approach is for a certain patient under specific circumstances. They can be categorized according to their clinical orientation (i.e., when the focus is on a specific process), their complexity, format (e.g., text vs. presented algorithms), clinical purpose (e.g., for screening, diagnosis, or treatment), and intended users (e.g., patients, doctors, nurses, or others).

Guidelines help healthcare providers make informed decisions when treating patients and choosing the most effective treatments. Patients can use guidelines to become active participants in their treatment by obtaining information about treatment options. Guidelines can reduce practice variations, healthcare costs, and deficiencies in clinical knowledge.

Treatment Manuals

Treatment manuals are used for easier implementation of clinical practice guidelines. Treatment manuals specify the content of guidelines and explain the practical aspects of guidelines. Treatment manuals have several advantages. Their time-limited and structured nature allows for a more highly focused treatment. They facilitate greater patient involvement in treatment. Treatment manuals can be used to train therapists in specific models, and they can reduce variability between practices.

However, treatment manuals have several disadvantages as well. They tend to involve mechanical implementation which makes them inflexible and nonintuitive. A treatment manual may not meet the patient's needs and may limit the healthcare provider merely the basics of what needs to be done. Treatment manuals may have a negative impact on the doctor-patient relationship.

Empirically Supported Treatments

Empirically supported treatments are an integration of the best available research combined with clinical experience. Empirically supported treatments have demonstrated effectiveness and achievement of positive outcomes in randomized controlled trials. There are many empirically supported treatments developed for mental health issues, such as cognitive behavioral therapy (CBT), or interpersonal psychotherapy. For example, multiple meta-analyses have shown that cognitive-behavioral therapy is a successful treatment for anxiety disorders and moderate or severe depression.

When using empirically supported treatments, clinicians should always view their judgment as a priority in the decision-making process. Clinicians should consider the individual patient's circumstances and the efficacy of empirically supported treatments for the condition they are treating. Clinicians should stay updated on the relevant literature, both in their area of interest and other areas.

Chapter 21: Legal and Ethical Considerations

Every healthcare provider is constantly faced with the challenge of making difficult decisions that can result in life or death. When caring for patients with mental health issues, complicated situations may arise. Healthcare providers are held to the highest standards of ethical and legal accountability in their practice. This chapter will discuss legal and ethical issues in psychiatry.

Medical Malpractice

Medical malpractice is a civil wrong that results from negligence. Negligence means that the clinician has done something that a clinician who has a duty to care for patients should not do, or they have not done something they should do, as defined by the current medical practice. To prove malpractice, the plaintiff (e.g., the patient or their family) should obtain evidence that: (1) there was a doctor-patient relationship, and the doctor had a duty to care for the patient (duty), (2) there was a deviation from the standard of care (deviation), (3) the patient was injured or damaged (damage), and (4) the deviation from the standard of care is what directly caused the damage (direct causation).

To find liability, each element of a malpractice claim should be present. For example, a psychiatrist cannot be liable for malpractice if there is no doctor-patient relationship that creates a duty of care, even if the psychiatrist's negligence causes direct harm to a patient. Psychiatrists are not liable if they advise on social media or television programs since there is no doctor-patient relationship in general advice-giving. Psychiatrists are not liable for malpractice if the patient's worsening condition is not related to negligence. Every bad outcome is not caused by negligence. Psychiatrists cannot guarantee that the diagnosis they have established is correct. Therefore, psychiatrists can make mistakes that cannot be defined as medical malpractice.

Other than negligence, patients can sue for false imprisonment, intentional tort of assault, defamation, battery, fraud, intentional infliction of emotional distress, and misrepresentation. Intentional tort means that the psychiatrist has done something that they realize, or should have realized, will bring harm to the patient.

Negligent Prescription Practices

Negligent prescription practice occurs when a clinician exceeds the recommended doses, does not adjust the medication levels to therapeutic, prescribes not-indicated medications, mixes medications unreasonably, does not disclose medication effects, or prescribes too many medications at the same time. Older patients take many medications prescribed by various physicians. When prescribing psychotropic medications, special care should be taken to avoid harmful interactions and side effects.

The prescribing clinician should document their reasons for prescribing multiple medications.

The prescribing clinician should explain to the patient the diagnosis they are receiving medication for, the risks, and the benefits of the drug. There is no consistently accepted standard for what information should be disclosed in a psychiatric or medical situation. Generally, the clinician should provide the patient with a description of their condition, the nature and goal of the proposed treatment, the risks and benefits of the treatment, possible alternatives to the treatment, their risks and benefits, and prognosis about the outcome with and without treatment.

Obtaining informed consent from a patient can be difficult if the patient has a reduced cognitive capacity due to mental illness or neurological disease. A substitute caretaker can provide consent in these situations. Informed consent should be obtained after every medication change or after introducing a new drug. If the doctor does not inform the patient of the risks associated with the medication and the medication injures the patient, there is sufficient ground for a malpractice claim.

Patients should be seen for medication follow-ups according to their needs. The follow-up interval should not go beyond six months. There is a higher likelihood of side effects and clinical developments with longer follow-up intervals. Psychiatrists may be sued for negligence if they fail to recognize and treat adverse effects or fail to monitor compliance with the limits of prescription. They may also be sued if they do not prescribe the appropriate amount of medication, or if they stop a medication inappropriately.

Split Treatment

Split treatment occurs when a psychiatrist prescribes medication, and another nonmedical therapist provides psychotherapy. Split treatment can cause fragmented care and may have dangerous consequences. The psychiatrist has the responsibility to be fully informed of the patient's status at all times. The psychiatrist should be informed of the quality and type of therapy the nonmedical therapist is providing. When the relationship between the psychiatrist and nonmedical therapist is collaborative, they both take responsibility for the patient's care. They should explain the different responsibilities of both providers to the patient. If the collaborative relationship ends, both parties should inform the patient about the termination.

Civil Rights of Patients

Least Restrictive Alternative

The least restrictive alternative principle states that patients should receive the least restrictive means of treatment necessary to achieve the desired outcome. If the patient can be treated as an outpatient, then they should not be committed. If the patient can be treated in an open ward, they should not be secluded.

Visitation Rights

Patients can receive visitors at the customary hospital visiting hours. There may be times when the patient's condition does not allow for visitations. If this is the case, the clinician should document the reasons. Certain visitors are not limited by visiting hours like the patient's private physician, the patient's attorney, or members of the clergy. However, in these situations, if the patient is in an emergency, even such visits can be limited. The patient's needs are always a priority.

Communication Rights

Open and free communication with the world outside is allowed, by phone or mail, but there may be exceptions to this case. In certain cases, jurisdictions charge hospitals with the duty to monitor the patients' communications. Patients with criminal charges of threatening or harassing phone calls should not be allowed unrestricted access to the phone. Patients are allowed to have private telephone calls, and the staff should not invade their privacy by listening to their conversations.

Economic Rights

Psychiatric patients are allowed to manage their finances, except in cases of incompetence. Patients should be paid if they work in the hospital (e.g., gardening, cooking).

Seclusion and Restraint

The U.S. Constitution protects every individual's security and privacy. According to the Bill of Rights for psychiatric patients, patients are free from restraint and seclusion, except in the case of emergencies. Seclusion and restraint have specific indications and contraindications. A patient can be secluded or restrained if they pose harm to themselves or others. Patients who are extremely unstable, delirious, demented, or overtly suicidal should not be secluded except if they are closely monitored and supervised. Only an appropriate medical official can give a written order for seclusion and restraint. It is strictly prohibited to use restraints as punishment or for the convenience of the staff. The condition of a secluded and restrained patient must be regularly observed, documented, and reviewed. Their vital signs, nutrition, elimination, and hydration should be assessed every ten to fifteen minutes.

Informed Consent

All patients have the right to decide what will happen or not happen to their bodies. Informed consent means that the patient has agreed to a specific treatment procedure after the healthcare provider has given enough information about the procedure, its risks, benefits, expected outcomes, and possible alternatives. In certain conditions, the patient's refusal of treatment can be dismissed. Examples include: when the patient is mentally incompetent to decide, the treatment is required to save their life or avoid severe harm, or if the refusal of treatment puts another's life or health in danger. In emergency situations, if the patient is not in a position to exercise judgment, the doctor does not have to obtain informed consent. If the patient is a child, his/her parents or surrogate are the ones who provide the consent. In the case of a therapeutic privilege, the clinician withholds information because full disclosure may complicate or obstruct treatment, be too upsetting for the patient, or cause severe psychological harm.

Most patients in psychiatric/mental health institutions can give informed consent. However, patients with severe psychiatric disorders often lack the cognitive capability to do so. If a patient is legally determined to be mentally incompetent, their legal guardian is the one who provides consent. In certain scenarios, a patient who is in a mental state that does not allow for informed decision-making (e.g., psychosis, unconsciousness), may not have a legal guardian. In these cases, consent should be obtained from the nearest relative. If the patient does not have a relative nearby, the clinician can ask the court to appoint a guardian.

Consent can be withdrawn at any time after it has been given. In these situations, the clinician should inform the patient or guardian about the consequences of rejecting treatment. The patient who signs an informed consent form should have: (1) knowledge and enough information to make an independent decision, (2) competency and cognition, and (3) free will – the patient must willingly sign the consent form without pressure from others.

Hospitalization

Informal Admission

The procedure of informal admission for psychiatric patients is the same as with other patients. The patient is free to leave and enter at any time, even if they are medically advised against it.

Voluntary Hospitalization

Voluntary hospitalization occurs when the patient applies on their own for admission to a psychiatric hospital. The patient is admitted if the examination finds that the patient needs hospital treatment. The patient is allowed to leave, even if they are medically advised against it.

Temporary Hospitalization

Patients who are senile, confused, or unable to make independent decisions and patients who are acutely disturbed and in need of immediate psychiatric treatment can be temporarily admitted to a psychiatric hospital. The hospital can admit the patient on the written recommendation of one clinician. Another psychiatrist or the hospital staff should confirm that the patient needs hospitalization, after admission. Temporary hospitalization usually lasts up to sixty days depending on state laws and regulations.

Involuntary Hospitalization

A person who is involuntarily hospitalized has significant restrictions on their rights of freedom. Involuntary hospitalization may be required when the patient is a danger to themself (suicidal) or others (homicidal), the patient needs observation or treatment, or if the patient is unable to take care of their basic personal needs. The individual who is seeking involuntary hospitalization must have sufficient evidence to show why the patient is being hospitalized against their will. Two doctors should examine the patient, and both should agree that the patient needs involuntary hospitalization.

Patients who are involuntarily hospitalized have the right to legal counsel. Their case can be brought before a judge. If the judge believes the patient should not be hospitalized, the patient is released. During the patient's stay, their case is reviewed periodically by a board that includes psychiatrists, lawyers, other physicians, and other citizens.

Types of Lawsuits in Psychiatric Nursing

Every hospitalized psychiatric patient has a right to privacy and confidentiality. The patient can sue the psychiatric nurse for breach of confidentiality if the nurse reveals details about their case or if he/she reveals that the patient has been hospitalized. Revealing that kind of sensitive information can result in harming the patient.

If shared information damages the patient's reputation, the person who shared the information can be liable for defamation of character. If the shared information is in written form, the liability is called libel. When the information is shared orally, it is called slander. Libel may occur when the patient's medical record contains critical or judgmental statements. Psychiatric nurses should back up everything they write in the chart with factual evidence.

If a patient is searched without probable cause, they can charge the institution with invasion of privacy. Routine body searches on psychiatric patients must be justified by a physician's order and should not be done without probable cause. In these situations, there should be a physician's order that states the reason for the body search.

Battery occurs when the patient is touched without consent. Battery may occur when the patient receives treatment against their wishes, in a non-emergency situation.

Chapter 22: Process Improvement

Quality and safety improvement initiatives are necessary in health care. A quality healthcare setting has a high likelihood of achieving desired health outcomes. Most medical errors occur due to imperfections in processes and systems, not individuals. Factors involved in the complexity of health care include inefficient processes, variability in health insurance, differences in education and experience of providers, variability in patient populations, and many others. A quality healthcare system should be safe, efficient, effective, timely, equitable, and patient-centered. Healthcare quality should be measured to assess the impact of healthcare on the desired outcomes and determine whether healthcare professionals adhere to processes that are based on scientific evidence and consistent with patient preferences.

Process improvement techniques should be implemented to identify potential inefficiencies, prevent potential errors or system failures, and improve care. Tools and strategies for improving the safety and quality of health care include Plan-Do-Study-Act, Lean, Six Sigma, root-cause analysis, failure modes, and effect analysis.

Quality Improvement Strategies

The quality of healthcare can be measured by assessing its structure, processes, and outcomes. The structure of healthcare determines the accessibility and availability of resources, as well as their quality. These include the number of nurses with appropriate education and training, the number of beds in the hospital, and health insurance. When measuring the process, assessment is done on the delivery of healthcare services by healthcare providers, such as the usage of up-to-date guidelines for the care of patients with anxiety disorders. The measurement of outcomes refers to the result of healthcare which is impacted by both behavioral and environmental factors. Outcomes include patient satisfaction, health status, morbidity, and mortality.

Continuous Quality Improvement

Continuous quality improvement (CQI) is used interchangeably with Total Quality Management (TQM). The CQI approach is based on the premise that to achieve the best outcome, the whole organization should commit to quality. It states that every process can be improved. The CQI approach is used to develop clinical practice. In-hospital quality assurance (QA) programs focus on problems identified by accreditation or regulatory organizations. These include a review of the work done by oversight committees, study of credentialing processes, and checking documentation.

Clinical practice improvement (CPI) is an approach that aims to implement change in the healthcare delivery process to achieve the best outcomes in the clinical management of patients. Quality improvement focuses on identification of processes that need to be improved. It then measures the factors involved in key performance, conducts a detailed analysis to develop a new approach, integrates the new approach with the process, and performs reassessments to determine whether the change has resulted in an improved process.

There are many strategies and tools that can be used to ensure quality improvement. Provide reminder systems through the incorporation of reminders in charts for providers, develop computer-based reminders and computer-based decision support. Provide audit and feedback by giving performance feedback to individual providers, incorporate quality indicators and reports, publicly release performance data, and incorporate National/State quality report cards. Educate providers by including them in workshops and conferences, distribute educational material and content, and initiate educational outreach visits. Educate patients by giving out patient pamphlets, include parents and families in the education process, and use education strategies that promote self-management of chronic disorders. Promote self-management by distributing postcards or calls to patients and develop patient reminder systems by giving materials and devices that promote self-management.

Plan-Do-Study-Act (PDSA)

The Plan-Do-Study-Act (PDSA) model aims to improve quality, make positive changes in healthcare, and achieve favorable outcomes. It is used for rapid cycle improvement. This model has a rapid cyclical nature and accomplishes change through regular and small PDSAs. The main purpose of PDSA is to demonstrate a relationship between process changes (e.g., behaviors and capabilities) and outcomes. Before using the PDSA cycles, three factors should be addressed: the goal of the project, how to know when the goal is reached, and what needs to be done to reach the goal.

Serious Reportable Adverse Events

Medical errors and failures in patient safety are an issue of health care quality. These occurrences are responsible for patient injury or death. The complexity and imperfection of the healthcare delivery system is responsible for the majority of medical lapses. Adverse events rarely occur because of negligence or medical malpractice.

Adverse events can be prevented through identification of the points in the healthcare process that are prone to mistakes and the implantation of changes to these processes in a way that will reduce the likelihood of harm. This requires obtaining data on preventable adverse events, which remain grossly underreported.

The Institute of Medicine (IOM) recommends systematic reporting of healthcare errors and adverse events to improve patient safety. The National Quality Forum (NQF) has identified a list of Serious Reportable Events in health care, referred to as the “never events.”

Purpose of the List of Serious Reportable Adverse Events

The main purpose of the list of serious reportable events was to identify a standard set of adverse events that would increase public accountability for their occurrence. This consensus list should represent a national state-based event reporting system that improves patient safety. Healthcare providers have public accountability to provide information about their performance and actions to the public. Oversight bodies exist to make sure that providers are compliant with accepted standards of care. When an adverse event occurs, oversight bodies should investigate the causes behind it. This information improves public safety.

Criteria of the List of Serious Reportable Adverse Events

The NQF list does not include all adverse events. For an event to be included in the list it must be measurable and identifiable, which makes it viable to be included in a standardized reporting system. The event's occurrence should be significantly influenced by the healthcare facility's procedures and policies. The event should pose a concern to the public and healthcare providers. The event should be serious, unambiguous, and preventable (in the majority of instances). It should indicate a problem in the safety systems of the healthcare facility, and it should have importance for public accountability or credibility.

The requirement that the event is preventable in the majority of instances, but not all instances, shows that not all events are preventable.

List of Serious Reportable Adverse Events

The list consists of twenty-seven serious reportable adverse events. They are organized in six categories. Five categories are related to the provision of care (e.g., care management, environmental, patient protection, product or device, and surgical), while one includes criminal events. Criminal events include acts of misconduct or illegal acts. The presence of criminal events indicates that the environment is unsafe for patients. Healthcare facilities are not able to fully eliminate the risk of adverse events. However, they can take actions and measures that will reduce that risk.

The list of serious reportable adverse events is short due to the belief that a clearly defined shortlist will be more easily understood and can be more widely used. The list can be seen on the NQF's website.

Chapter 23: Outcome Measurement

Psychiatric Rating Scales

Psychiatric rating scales include questionnaires, checklists, outcome assessments, and other instruments that are used to inform psychiatric practice, research, and administration. Mental health providers should use psychiatric rating scales for several reasons. Psychiatric rating scales can be used to monitor the patient's progress over time. They can provide more information than a routine clinical interview. Healthcare administrators, insurance companies, and other stakeholders might require standardized assessments in order to assess the quality of care and the need for mental health services. Psychiatric rating scales are used in research. By understanding them, the clinician can obtain more knowledge from that research and lead an evidence-based practice. The use of validated rating scales is necessary for measurement-based practice.

Benefits of Psychiatric Rating Scales

The main goal of psychiatric rating scales is to standardize information about the patient that has been collected by various providers. By standardizing information, healthcare providers can have a comprehensive evaluation which can be used as an aid in treatment planning. Psychiatric rating scales can help clinicians establish an accurate diagnosis, thoroughly describe symptoms, identify any potential comorbid conditions, and assess factors that impact treatment response. A rating scale can establish a baseline that will be used to monitor the progression of a disorder over time or in response to therapeutic interventions. This can be especially useful when multiple providers are caring for the patient, for example, in a group practice.

Types of Scales and What They Measure

Psychiatric rating scales can achieve many different goals. They can cover a broad range of areas and can be used in various formats.

Measurement Goals

Psychiatric rating scales can be most commonly categorized into scales that are used to make a diagnosis, scales for measuring the severity of symptoms and tracking changes in the severity of the specific symptoms, scales for monitoring change in general functioning or overall outcome, and scales that screen for other conditions.

Constructs Assessed

The broad ranges of areas that scales assess are referred to as constructs. Constructs can be diagnoses, quality of life, functional impairment, severity, signs, symptoms, etc. Some constructs are complex and need to be divided into a few domains, for example, positive and negative symptoms of schizophrenia.

Constructs can be categorical (or classifying), continuous, or measuring. Categorical constructs are used to describe whether a feature is currently present or absent (e.g., the ability to work a full-time job) or the category to which the patient belongs among other options (e.g., establishing a diagnosis). Continuous scales are used to provide a quantitative assessment (measurement) of severity, frequency, or intensity. Continuous scales can measure cognitive status, multidimensional personality traits, symptom severity, functional status, and others.

Measurement Methods

Rating scales use different measuring methods. They differ in format, raters, and sources of information.

Format

Scales are available in many formats that include checklists, self-administered questionnaires, tests, guides to observation, etc. Some scales are fully structured formal interviews. In a fully structured formal interview, the exact wordings of the questions that are asked are specified. Scales can be in the form of partially structured interviews which require only some specific wording, and additional questions or statements are allowed.

Raters

Some psychiatric rating instruments are designed to be used only by doctoral-level clinicians. Some rating scales can be administered by social workers with clinical experience or psychiatric nurses. Other scales are designed for the layperson without clinical experience or knowledge of psychopathology.

Source of Information

Instruments can obtain information from different sources. The patient who fully understands his/her condition can be the only source of information. In some situations, the use of an informant is preferable. For example, when the patient has limited insight into their condition (e.g., psychosis or mania), or if the patient has severe social undesirability (e.g., antisocial personality disorder or substance use disorder), it is better to use other informants to obtain information. Another situation that can benefit from the use of an informant is when the patient is unable to recall or report symptoms (e.g., cognitive disorder, delirium, dementia, or disorders in young children). Some instruments require information that can only be obtained from medical records or direct patient observation.

Selection of Psychiatric Rating Scales

Many scales can be used in clinical practice. Explaining all of them is beyond the scope of this chapter. Here we will discuss the most used rating scales that cover areas such as symptom severity, diagnosis, functioning, and others.

Disability Assessment

The World Health Organization developed the WHO Disability Assessment Schedule scale, the most commonly used scale to measure disability. It is now in its second edition (WHODAS 2.0). This scale is self-administered and measures several parameters of disability like interpersonal relations, work impairment, social impairment, cognition, etc. The WHODAS 2.0 can be administered at different intervals throughout the illness. It can track changes that occur as a positive or negative response to a therapeutic intervention.

Psychotic Disorders

Many instruments are used for patients with psychotic disorders. Most scales are designed to monitor treatment effects in clinical research. In psychotic disorder, the patient has limited insight, therefore scales often require information from informants or clinicians.

Positive and Negative Syndrome Scale (PANSS)

The PANNS is used to assess positive and negative symptoms of schizophrenia and other psychotic disorders. It is designed for clinicians since it requires clinical judgment. There is a semi-structured interview guide developed for this scale. The PANNS is the gold standard instrument for assessing clinical outcomes in studies of schizophrenia treatment. It can also be used to track symptom severity in clinical settings.

Mood Disorders

Instruments that are used in the domain of mood disorders assess depression and mania. Patients who are in mania have limited insight, while agitation may impair the ability to accurately report symptoms. Therefore, rating scales generally require clinician ratings and data obtained from informants. Depression, however, depends on the patient's subjective experience of their mood state. Interview and self-reporting scales are common in the assessment of depression. Because of the high prevalence of depression, and its significant morbidity and mortality, it is important to incorporate screening instruments in primary care and community settings.

Hamilton Rating Scale for Depression (HAM-D)

The HAM-D is used to measure the symptom severity of major depression, with a focus on somatic complaints. There are versions with different numbers of items, but the most used one is the seventeen-item version. The HAM-D was originally developed for clinician raters, but it is not usually used by lay administrators. The ratings are completed by the person who is interviewing with the patient and are based on their observations. There is a structured interview guide that can improve reliability. The HAM-D can assess changes in response to health interventions (e.g., pharmacological interventions). It may be problematic to use in elderly patients and patients with medical illnesses since the presence of somatic symptoms in these patients may not be a sign of major depression.

Beck Depression Inventory (BDI)

The BDI measures depression severity. It focuses on the cognitive and behavioral dimensions of depression. The BDI-II (current version) includes somatic symptoms and focuses on the most recent two weeks. Previous versions focus on shorter intervals. The BDI is a self-report instrument that can be completed in five to ten minutes. Its main use is a measurement of outcomes in studies for major depression interventions. The BDI can be used as a screening instrument for major depression.

Anxiety Disorders

Anxiety disorders rating scales can be interviews or self-report rating scales. The measures depend on the patient's subjective experience of their inner state.

Hamilton Anxiety Rating Scale (HAM-A)

The HAM-A assesses somatic and cognitive symptoms of anxiety. It should be administered by a clinician. A structured interview guide is available to achieve high reliability. The HAM-A can be used to monitor the treatment response of GAD in clinical settings and clinical practice.

Panic Disorder Severity Scale (PDSS)

The PDSS measures the severity of panic disorder. It consists of seven items that measure the frequency of panic attacks, the distress associated with attacks, phobic avoidance, anticipatory anxiety, and impairment. It can be used to monitor panic disorder in clinical practice and to measure outcomes in clinical trials.

Clinician-Administered PTSD Scale (CAPS)

The CAPS consist of thirty items that cover all DSM-5 criteria for PTSD (the original traumatic event, reexperiencing of the event, avoidance, negative alterations in cognitions and mood, and increased arousal). It is used to establish the diagnosis of PTSD. The CAPS also includes global rating scales that measure the impact PTSD has on the patient's social and occupational functioning. The CAPS is designed to be administered by a trained clinician. It takes forty-five to ninety minutes to be completed. It is used in clinical studies for diagnosis and severity assessment. Because of its length, it is not convenient to use in clinical practice.

Yale-Brown Obsessive-Compulsive Scale (YBOCS)

The YBOCS is a rating scale that measures the severity of OCD symptoms. It consists of ten items. The first five items are related to obsessions: how much time they consume, to what degree they interfere in the patient's daily functioning, how much distress they cause, how much the patient attempts to resist, and how the patient is able to control them. The other five items are parallel questions about compulsions. The YBOCS is completed in ten to fifteen minutes. It can be used to assess OCD severity in treatment studies as well as in clinical practice to monitor treatment response.

Substance Use Disorders

CAGE

The CAGE is a short screening instrument for alcohol problems that can be used in various settings. CAGE is an acronym for four questions. A score of one is given to each answer "yes." A score of one means the person might have an alcohol problem and needs to be followed up. A score of two or more suggests significant alcohol problems. The instrument can be completed in less than one minute.

Addiction Severity Index (ASI)

The ASI measures symptoms and functional impairment caused by drug or alcohol abuse. It consists of demographics, drug use, alcohol use, medical status, psychiatric status, employment, family issues, social issues, and legal status. The ASI assesses the duration, frequency, and severity of drug or alcohol use. Both subjective and objective reports by the patient and the interviewer are included.

Cognitive Disorders

Mini-Mental State Examination (MMSE)

The MMSE is a cognitive test that consists of thirty points. It is used to assess cognitive functions in many domains (orientation, memory, language, attention, and construction). The MMSE has excellent reliability and good validity.

Neuropsychiatric Inventory (NPI)

The NPI is used to assess behavioral symptoms seen in Alzheimer's disease and other types of dementia. It assesses twelve areas: apathy, aberrant motor behavior, appetite, anxiety, agitation/aggression, delusions, dysphoria, disinhibition, euphoria, irritability/lability, nocturnal disturbances, and eating. The NPI is an interview that is performed by a trained interviewer or a clinician with a caregiver or other informant. It can be completed in fifteen to twenty minutes. There is a version for a nursing home interview (NPI-NH), and a self-report questionnaire (NPI-Q). For every area, the NPI first asks if the symptom is present. If the answer is yes, then it assesses the severity, frequency, and the caregiver's distress. The NPI is used in both research and clinical settings.

Scored General Intelligence Test (SGIT)

The SGIT test measures general intelligence. The clinician can administer the SGIT during a psychiatric interview. Any decline in general intelligence can be a sign of a cognitive disorder and requires further work-up.

Test 1: Questions

(1) The successful resolution of the crisis in each of Erikson's stages of psychosocial development leads to:

(A) The development of a maladaptive personality.

(B) The development of a healthy personality.

(C) The development of an insecure attachment style.

(D) The development of an anxious-ambivalent attachment style.

(2) What is the main conflict in the first stage of psychosocial development?

(A) Trust versus mistrust.

(B) Autonomy versus shame and doubt.

(C) Industry versus inferiority.

(D) Initiative versus guilt.

(3) What are the consequences of an unsuccessful resolution of the first stage of psychosocial development?

(A) The infant doubts its abilities.

(B) The infant is not able to explore its interests.

(C) The infant is not able to form secure attachments.

(D) The infant does not trust the world.

(4) Children develop autonomy and independence during the:

(A) First stage of psychosocial development.

(B) Fourth stage of psychosocial development.

(C) Second stage of psychosocial development.

(D) Third stage of psychosocial development.

(5) Which of the following statements is true about the second stage of psychosocial development?

(A) If parents successfully encourage their children's independence, the children will develop self-confidence and autonomy.

(B) If the parents do not provide security, comfort, care, and affection, an infant will develop mistrust.

(C) The basic virtue acquired during the second stage of psychosocial development is hope.

(D) The basic virtue acquired during the second stage of psychosocial development is trust.

(6) Initiative versus guilt is the major conflict in the:

(A) First stage of psychosocial development.

(B) Fourth stage of psychosocial development.

(C) Second stage of psychosocial development.

(D) Third stage of psychosocial development.

(7) A four-year-old child asks his father, "Why don't birds live in human houses?" His father is immersed in a movie and becomes annoyed that the child interrupted him. He answers, "Don't ask me such stupid questions!" How might this response affect the child's psychosocial development?

(A) It will help him develop industry instead of inferiority.

(B) It might cause guilt, which can damage the child's curiosity and creativity.

(C) It will create a healthy personality.

(D) It will help him develop independence.

(8) Industry versus inferiority is the major conflict in the:

(A) First stage of psychosocial development.

(B) Fourth stage of psychosocial development.

(C) Second stage of psychosocial development.

(D) Third stage of psychosocial development.

(9) Which of the following statements is false about the fourth stage of psychosocial development?

(A) The social component is developed during the fourth stage of psychosocial development.

(B) Children start to develop interests in things such as sports, music, art, etc.

(C) Parents and teachers expect children to perform well in elementary school.

(D) The basic conflict in this stage is initiative versus guilt.

(10) The transition from childhood to adulthood is the:

(A) First stage of psychosocial development.

(B) Fourth stage of psychosocial development.

(C) Fifth stage of psychosocial development.

(D) Third stage of psychosocial development.

(11) Which of the following interventions is most effective for improving sleep modulation for patients with chronic insomnia?

(A) Increasing daytime napping.

(B) Implementing a strict bedtime routine.

(C) Encouraging the use of sleep medications.

(D) Allowing variable sleep and wake times.

(12) According to Erik Erikson, role confusion during the fifth stage of psychosocial development is:

(A) A normal occurrence.

(B) A maladaptive occurrence.

(C) A sign of failed resolution.

(D) A sign of unhealthy characteristics.

(13) A 17-year-old girl has expressed the wish to go to drama school. Her parents are very angry. They own a cardiovascular practice, and they always planned that their daughter would be a cardiologist who would expand the family business. What kind of advice should the mental health nurse practitioner offer the parents?

(A) Parents should allow their children to develop their own identity.

(B) The family business is more important than the daughter's future plans.

(C) Parents should always make life decisions for their children since they are older and have more life experience.

(D) They should not take their daughter's wish seriously since it is most likely a phase.

(14) What are the consequences of an unsuccessful resolution of the fifth stage of psychosocial development?

(A) A meaningless life causes stagnation and disconnection from the community and society.

(B) A failure to develop close relationships can cause isolation, loneliness, and depression.

(C) Unresolved identity issues leave a person confused about their direction in life and role in society.

(D) Too much criticism causes low self-esteem and doubt about one's capabilities.

(15) What is the sixth stage of Erik Erikson's psychological development?

(A) Trust vs. Mistrust.

(B) Autonomy vs. Shame and Doubt.

(C) Intimacy vs. Isolation.

(D) Integrity vs. Despair.

(16) Individuals who are in the seventh stage of psychosocial development are likely to:

(A) Develop an intimate relationship with another person who is not a family member.

(B) Learn to trust their capabilities.

(C) Consider what they have left behind for their community.

(D) Wonder whether the world is a trustworthy or a dangerous place.

(17) Which of the following statements is false about the seventh stage of psychosocial development?

(A) If a person has failed to work toward a meaningful goal, they will feel stagnation and emptiness.

(B) The successful resolution of this stage leads to the development of the virtue of care.

(C) Parenthood is a significant task during this part of life.

(D) Adults who don't achieve generativity feel connected to their community.

(18) Individuals who are in the seventh stage of psychosocial development:

(A) Interact and play with other children.

(B) Find a partner to start a family.

(C) Contemplate college choices.

(D) Create and maintain a comfortable home.

(19) What happens in the eighth stage of psychosocial development?

(A) People retire and have more time to reflect on their lives.

(B) People develop their identity.

(C) People build productive careers.

(D) People try to become better versions of themselves.

(20) The basic conflict in the eighth stage is:

(A) Generativity versus stagnation.

(B) Intimacy versus isolation.

(C) Identity versus role confusion.

(D) Ego integrity versus despair.

(21) A female patient, 27 years of age, complains of depressed mood, fatigue, loss of interest in activities that used to bring her pleasure, memory loss, and an irregular menstrual cycle. Upon physical examination, you notice that she has dry skin and is inappropriately dressed. What is the next diagnostic test the psychiatric mental health nurse practitioner should order?

(A) Alkaline phosphatase levels.

(B) Thyroid function tests.

(C) Liver function tests.

(D) Magnetic resonance imaging.

(22) A patient presents with increased anxiety and panic attacks. He complains that he sweats excessively and can feel his heartbeat is very fast. In the past month, he has lost six pounds. Which diagnosis should the psychiatric mental health nurse practitioner suspect?

(A) Systemic lupus erythematosus.

(B) Schizophrenia.

(C) Graves's disease.

(D) Hypothyroidism.

(23) An endocrinologic disease is characterized by elevated cortisol levels, thin atrophic skin, increased appetite, irregularities of the menstrual cycle, hypercholesterolemia, hypertriglyceridemia, glucose intolerance, hirsutism, fat redistribution, dysphoria, irritability, insomnia, cognitive impairment (memory loss, inattention, problems with concentration), depressive and manic symptoms, and in some cases, psychotic episodes. What is this disease called?

(A) Graves's disease.

(B) Cushing's syndrome.

(C) Addison's disease.

(D) Hashimoto's thyroiditis.

(24) A patient diagnosed with major depressive disorder complains of fatigue, diarrhea, loss of appetite, and an increased need for salt. What test should the psychiatric mental health nurse practitioner order?

(A) Estrogen levels.

(B) A CT of the abdomen.

(C) MRI of the brain.

(D) Serum cortisol and ACTH measurement.

(25) Which vitamin deficiency causes the triad of ataxia, cognitive deficiencies in attention and orientation, and oculomotor dysfunction?

(A) Vitamin B1 deficiency

(B) Vitamin C deficiency.

(C) Vitamin B12 deficiency.

(D) Vitamin D deficiency.

(26) A 65-year-old patient who had a prior small bowel resection complains of depression, memory loss, pins and needles in her legs, and urinary incontinence. The psychiatric mental health nurse practitioner should:

(A) Order liver function tests.

(B) Order serum vitamin B12 tests.

(C) Interpret the symptoms as a part of major depressive disorder.

(D) Suspect that the patient has a somatoform disorder.

(27) Which of the following statements is false about calcium levels and neuropsychiatric symptoms?

(A) Neuropsychiatric symptoms can occur as a result of elevated or decreased calcium levels in the blood.

(B) Hypocalcemia causes seizures, disorientation, confusion, emotional lability, delirium, anxiety, depression, and psychosis.

(C) Hypercalcemia causes confusion, weakness, lethargy, drowsiness, and depressive symptoms.

(D) Hypocalcemia is not associated with psychiatric symptoms.

(28) A patient with bipolar disorder type I suffers from confusion and lethargy. Physical examination is unremarkable. Laboratory tests show elevated calcium levels. Which medications could be responsible for the development of hypercalcemia?

(A) Fluoxetine.

(B) Lamotrigine.

(C) Risperidone.

(D) Lithium.

(29) An autosomal recessive disorder that affects the hepatic transport of copper and causes neuropsychiatric symptoms is:

(A) Wilson's disease.

(B) Systemic lupus erythematosus.

(C) Porphyria.

(D) Graves's disease.

(30) A 14-year-old patient is hospitalized because of aggressive behavior, cognitive impairment, and disinhibition. The patient presents with ataxia and, on ophthalmologic slit-lamp examination, has a Kayser-Fleischer ring. What is the next step in the management of this patient?

(A) Order serum ACTH measurement.

(B) Order 24-hour urine copper quantification.

(C) Administer intravenous olanzapine.

(D) Administer intramuscular diazepam.

(31) A systemic autoimmune disease characterized by the presence of autoantibodies directed against neuronal membranes and antibodies against NMDA receptors that cause psychiatric symptoms like depression, mood disorders, anxiety disorders, psychosis, and cognitive decline is:

(A) Hashimoto's thyroiditis.

(B) Addison's disease.

(C) Systemic lupus erythematosus.

(D) Sarcoidosis.

(32) A patient who suffers from systemic lupus erythematosus develops hallucinations and delusions. Which of the following statements is correct about this patient's condition?

(A) The patient has developed psychosis because of treatment with azathioprine.

(B) The patient has developed psychosis because of treatment with cyclophosphamide.

(C) The patient has developed psychosis because of his disease.

(D) The patient might have developed psychosis either because of his disease or because of treatment with corticosteroids.

(33) A 40-year-old patient complains of chest pain. He is diagnosed with esophageal dysmotility. Which of the following psychiatric disorders that can be comorbid with this condition should the psychiatric mental health nurse practitioner suspect?

(A) Schizophrenia.

(B) Bipolar disorder type I.

(C) Generalized anxiety disorder.

(D) Obsessive-compulsive disorder.

(34) Which of the following statements is false about the association between irritable bowel syndrome and psychiatric symptoms?

(A) Emotional stress causes increased sympathetic nervous system activity, which causes inhibition of gastric motility.

(B) Psychiatric disorders are frequently found in patients who suffer from IBS.

(C) The most common psychiatric disorders found in patients with irritable bowel syndrome are panic disorder, social phobia, generalized anxiety disorder, and major depressive disorder.

(D) The most common psychiatric disorders found in patients with irritable bowel syndrome are schizophrenia, schizoaffective disorder, and OCD.

(35) A patient previously diagnosed with irritable bowel syndrome and depression complains of increased frequency of stools. Which medications can be beneficial for both mood and gastrointestinal symptoms?

(A) Selective serotonin reuptake inhibitors.

(B) Selective noradrenaline reuptake inhibitors.

(C) Second-generation antipsychotics.

(D) Tricyclic antidepressants.

(36) A 67-year-old COPD patient with a smoking history of 45 years complains of frequent panic attacks. On physical examination, there is lung overinflation, use of accessory muscles that help with respiration, wheezing on auscultation, and diminished breath sounds. Which medications should the psychiatric mental health nurse practitioner avoid for the treatment of this man's panic attacks?

(A) Diazepam.

(B) Haloperidol.

(C) Chlorpromazine.

(D) Fluphenazine.

(37) What is the most common psychiatric disorder associated with gastroesophageal reflux disease?

(A) Anxiety disorder.

(B) Schizophrenia.

(C) Major depressive disorder.

(D) Dissociative identity disorder.

(38) Which of the following statements is correct about COPD patients and psychiatric symptoms?

(A) Persecutory delusions are the most common psychotic symptom seen in patients with COPD.

(B) Ideas of reference are the most common psychiatric symptom seen in patients with COPD.

(C) Psychiatric symptoms seen in patients with COPD may be due to chronic hypoxia or treatment with corticosteroid medications.

(D) Benzodiazepines are the medication of choice for patients with COPD who have panic attacks.

(39) A 35-year-old patient presents with chronic fatigue, depressive mood, irritability, and excessive daytime sleepiness. The psychiatric mental health nurse practitioner should screen for:

(A) Bipolar Disorder Type II.

(B) Adverse childhood experience (ACE) score.

(C) Chronic obstructive pulmonary disease.

(D) Obstructive sleep apnea.

(40) During the interview, you ask the patient to describe herself. She reports that she is a very ambitious person who never gets sad and can face any challenge life throws at her. She works multiple jobs and looks down on people who "waste their lives by watching TV." She complains that sometimes she gets very angry easily, especially because of other people's failures. She is frequently worried about having a physical illness. What is this patient at risk for?

(A) Systemic lupus erythematosus.

(B) Cardiac morbidity or mortality.

(C) Chronic obstructive pulmonary disease.

(D) Obstructive sleep apnea.

(41) Which of the following statements is false about schizophrenia?

(A) Schizophrenia is characterized by the inability of the patient to test reality.

(B) Schizophrenia is a severe mental disorder that causes significant long-lasting impairments and disability.

(C) Schizophrenia causes impairments in perception, cognition, emotion, behavior, eye movement, and socialization.

(D) Women tend to have more negative symptoms compared to men.

(42) Which type of hallucinations are most common in schizophrenia?

(A) Olfactory hallucinations.

(B) Auditory hallucinations.

(C) Gustatory hallucinations.

(D) Visual hallucinations.

(43) A male patient in his twenties presents to the emergency room, shouting that he is the messiah sent by God and his purpose is to save the world. He is agitated, and it is very difficult to understand his words. He constantly talks to himself. What is the most likely diagnosis?

(A) Bipolar disorder.

(B) Psychosis.

(C) Panic attack.

(D) Depressive episode.

(44) Which of the following statements is false about affective symptoms of schizophrenia?

(A) Patients with schizophrenia may present with anhedonia.

(B) Patients with schizophrenia often have a flat or blunted affect.

(C) Patients with schizophrenia may present with extreme rage.

(D) The hallmark of schizophrenia is an elevated, expansive, grandiose mood.

(45) What are the positive symptoms of schizophrenia?

(A) Hallucinations, delusions, and disorganized, bizarre behaviors.

(B) Blunted affect, absence of motivation, pleasure, attention, and thought.

(C) Impairment in attention, episodic memory, working memory, and executive function.

(D) Anhedonia, depression, anxiety, extreme rage.

(46) A female patient, 35 years of age, presents to the emergency department accompanied by her family. Her sister reports that in the past two weeks, the patient has acted very unusually. She has gotten into fights with family members, spent nearly all her savings on a shopping spree, and appears to have a lot of energy and no need for sleep. When you examine the patient, you notice she is irritated and talks very fast, with a sense of urgency. What is the most likely diagnosis?

(A) Panic disorder.

(B) Manic episode.

(C) Psychotic episode.

(D) Hypomanic episode.

(47) A male patient, 39 years old, complains that he feels numb and has lost interest in his hobbies in the past month. He reports he eats very little but does not feel hungry, and he has trouble falling asleep. What is the most likely diagnosis?

(A) Panic disorder.

(B) Schizophrenia.

(C) Major depressive disorder.

(D) Bipolar disorder.

(48) What is a less severe type of major depressive disorder?

(A) Cyclothymia.

(B) Dysthymia.

(C) Depression with psychotic features.

(D) Seasonal depression.

(49) What is the definition of a neurocognitive disorder?

(A) Neurocognitive disorders are caused by a medical or neurological condition that manifests as psychiatric and/or neurologic symptomatology and changes in cognition.

(B) Neurocognitive disorders are characterized by a short-term decline in consciousness and cognition.

(C) Neurocognitive disorders are characterized by a progressive decline of cognitive abilities in the setting of a clear consciousness.

(D) Neurocognitive disorders are characterized by the patient's inability to test reality.

(50) A neurocognitive disorder with an acute onset characterized by a short-term decline in consciousness and cognition is called:

(A) Dementia.

(B) Delirium.

(C) Alzheimer's disease.

(D) Huntington's disease.

(51) A neurocognitive disorder characterized by a progressive decline of cognitive abilities in the setting of a clear consciousness is called:

(A) Dementia.

(B) Delirium.

(C) Alzheimer's disease.

(D) Huntington's disease.

(52) A personality disorder that is characterized by excessive suspiciousness of others is called:

(A) Paranoid personality disorder.

(B) Avoidant personality disorder.

(C) Antisocial personality disorder.

(D) Schizoid personality disorder.

(53) A patient who is hospitalized because of major depressive disorder tells the other patients she can read their minds and communicate with people from her past life. On examination, there are no signs of perceptual disturbances and psychosis. The psychiatric mental health nurse practitioner suspects:

(A) Paranoid personality disorder.

(B) Schizotypal personality disorder.

(C) Antisocial personality disorder.

(D) Schizoid personality disorder.

(54) A personality disorder characterized by a pervasive disrespect for other people's rights is called:

(A) Borderline personality disorder.

(B) Dependent personality disorder.

(C) Antisocial personality disorder.

(D) Schizoid personality disorder.

(55) Which of the following statements is true about borderline personality disorder (BPD)?

(A) Patients with BPD have an intense fear of abandonment.

(B) Patients with BPD disrespect others' rights.

(C) Patients with BPD can be manipulative.

(D) Patients with BPD have no remorse for their actions.

(56) Which personality disorder is characterized by an exaggerated sense of self-importance and grandiosity?

(A) Avoidant personality disorder.

(B) Schizoid personality disorder.

(C) Paranoid personality disorder.

(D) Narcissistic personality disorder.

(57) Which personality disorder is not a part of cluster C (anxious) personality disorders?

(A) Avoidant personality disorder.

(B) Dependent personality disorder.

(C) Obsessive-compulsive personality disorder.

(D) Schizotypal personality disorder.

(58) Patients with anxiety often have:

(A) Superstitious beliefs.

(B) Ruminations about potential dangers.

(C) Beliefs of magical powers.

(D) Beliefs of grandiosity.

(59) A type of anxiety disorder characterized by a fear of situations or places that might be difficult to escape is called:

(A) Specific phobia.

(B) Generalized anxiety disorder.

(C) Agoraphobia.

(D) Panic disorder.

(60) What is a set of behaviors a person uses to deal with stress?

(A) Flexible behaviors.

(B) Adaptive behaviors.

(C) Coping styles.

(D) Defense mechanisms.

(61) Which of the following statements is incorrect about coping and defense mechanisms?

(A) Defense mechanisms are involuntary subconscious adaptive coping mechanisms that warp one's perception of reality.

(B) Defense mechanisms can reduce a person's feelings of anxiety, depression, and distress.

(C) Coping mechanisms are thoughts and behaviors that can be used to overcome or manage stressful situations.

(D) Problem-focused coping is characterized by the search for a higher meaning from the situation that might improve one's life in the future.

(62) Excessive use of defensive mechanisms might cause:

(A) Resolution of the stressful situation.

(B) Psychopathology and neuroses.

(C) Increased cardiovascular morbidity and mortality.

(D) Dissociative experiences.

(63) A 40-year-old female patient who lost her son in a car accident says he called her yesterday and asked her to buy groceries. She refuses to believe her son is gone, and she insists he is waiting for her at home. Which coping mechanism is the patient using?

(A) Denial.

(B) Repression.

(C) Dissociation.

(D) Projection.

(64) A patient is very critical of the appearance of staff members. He comments on their clothes, weight, the color of their hair, etc. In a conversation, the patient admits he sometimes feels insecure about the way he looks. Which coping mechanism is this patient using?

(A) Regression.

(B) Repression.

(C) Dissociation.

(D) Projection.

(65) A patient is going through a divorce. You notice she has started to suck her thumb. She says she hasn't done that in years, but it used to be a bad habit. Which coping mechanism is this patient using?

(A) Conversion.

(B) Introjection.

(C) Dissociation.

(D) Regression.

(66) Jim, a 22-year-old student, is about to graduate. After he graduates, he plans to go back to his hometown and find a job. He and his girlfriend will have to be in a long-distance relationship since she has a year left at university. Jim is confident that their relationship will survive and says he does not feel any anxiety. He reports that in the past six months, he has had weird pains all over his body. He has gone to many doctors, and all the tests have returned normal results. Which defense mechanism is Jim using?

(A) Conversion.

(B) Introjection.

(C) Dissociation.

(D) Regression.

(67) Caroline is a very successful woman who complains of feelings of unworthiness. When Caroline was a child, her mother had very high expectations of her, and she criticized her if she failed to live up to them. Caroline always struggled with her low self-esteem, and she compensated by working too hard. Which defense mechanism did Caroline develop as a child?

(A) Splitting.

(B) Introjection.

(C) Identification with the aggressor.

(D) Dissociation.

(68) A defense mechanism that occurs when a victim adopts the behavior of an aggressor as an attempt to avoid abuse and induce empathy is:

(A) Conversion.

(B) Introjection.

(C) Projection.

(D) Identification with the aggressor.

(69) Jennifer and Claire are very close friends. Claire is always there for Jennifer when she needs her, and Jennifer believes that Claire is the best person in the world. When Jennifer asks Claire to go to the theater one night, Claire turns her down because she has a lot of work to do. Jennifer gets mad and calls her selfish and unreliable. At that moment, Jennifer is unable to recognize all the times that Claire has been a good friend. Which defense mechanism has Jennifer developed?

(A) Jennifer has developed splitting.

(B) Jennifer has developed projection.

(C) Jennifer has developed conversion.

(D) Jennifer has developed repression.

(70) A defense mechanism characterized by blocking undesirable and uncomfortable feelings, ideas, memories, or impulses is called:

(A) Conversion.

(B) Introjection.

(C) Projection.

(D) Repression.

(71) Harry is under a lot of stress. In the past year, he has dealt with worsening mental health and his mother's diagnosis with dementia. He has no savings left, and his boss threatens to fire him because he is unfocused at work. In order to forget about these events, Harry immerses himself in fantasies about a perfect life. Sometimes, he fantasizes for hours. Which defense mechanism is Harry using?

(A) Undoing.

(B) Splitting.

(C) Dissociation.

(D) Regression.

(72) Which of the following is a higher-level defense mechanism?

(A) Splitting.

(B) Projection.

(C) Dissociation.

(D) Anticipation.

(73) Which of the following best describes the defense mechanism of compensation?

(A) Redirecting emotions from a threatening object to a safer one.

(B) Refusing to acknowledge an aspect of reality.

(C) Channeling unacceptable impulses into socially acceptable activities.

(D) Overcoming perceived weaknesses by emphasizing strengths in other areas.

(74) Marie is angry because she got stopped by the police for speeding. She behaves very calmly with the policeman. When she comes home, she yells at her dog. Which defense mechanism is Marie using?

(A) Displacement.

(B) Humor.

(C) Splitting.

(D) Reaction formation.

(75) Adam went to the grocery store to buy his favorite chocolate. When he got there, he realized they were out of stock. He bought another brand and said to himself, "I wanted to try another one either way." Which defense mechanism is Adam using?

(A) Reaction formation.

(B) Intellectualization.

(C) Humor.

(D) Rationalization.

(76) A 10-year-old boy has a crush on a girl from his class. He is too shy to talk to her, so he pulls her hair instead. Which defense mechanism is this?

(A) Reaction formation.

(B) Intellectualization.

(C) Humor.

(D) Rationalization.

(77) The doctor informs Beth that she has cervical cancer. Beth does not show any sadness when she hears the bad news. When she goes home, she starts to research cervical cancer. Which defense mechanism is Beth using?

(A) Displacement.

(B) Reaction formation.

(C) Sublimation.

(D) Intellectualization

(78) Derrick gets into an argument with his friend. The argument gets heated, and he has an urge to hit his friend. Instead, Derrick goes for a jog. Which defense mechanism is this?

(A) Repression.

(B) Suppression.

(C) Sublimation.

(D) Reaction formation.

(79) A patient with BPD has a history of sexual abuse. She complains that she frequently has intrusive thoughts about the event, but she blocks them in order to function in her daily life. Which defense mechanism is this?

(A) Repression.

(B) Suppression.

(C) Splitting.

(D) Displacement.

(80) What is the first part of the psychiatric interview?

(A) Perceptual disturbance.

(B) Mental state examination.

(C) Trauma history.

(D) Basic information about the patient.

(81) The chronological description of the course of a patient's symptoms is called:

(A) Past psychiatric history.

(B) Family history.

(C) History of present illness.

(D) Chief complaint.

(82) In order to get information about previous psychiatric diseases in a new patient, the psychiatric mental health nurse practitioner should:

(A) Order a list of medications.

(B) Ask the patient to fill out a dissociative experiences scale.

(C) Take a detailed past psychiatric history.

(D) Order a complete blood count.

(83) When she asks a patient about substance use, the psychiatric mental health nurse practitioner should:

(A) Use a nonjudgmental manner in order to obtain accurate information.

(B) Ask the patient to stop the substance use if she wants the treatment to be successful.

(C) Ignore the substance use and ask about family problems.

(D) Ask the patient how she finds illegal substances.

(84) Which of the following statements is false about past medical history and psychiatric disease?

(A) A medical condition can worsen the symptoms of a psychiatric illness, such as when a patient with anxiety is diagnosed with cancer.

(B) A medical condition cannot be precipitated by the treatment of a psychiatric illness.

(C) Past medical history is an essential part of the psychiatric interview.

(D) Past medical history should include the presence of any medical conditions, surgical history, and treatment.

(85) In order to assess the patient's capacity to develop and maintain interpersonal relationships, the psychiatric mental health nurse practitioner should ask about:

(A) School history.

(B) Developmental history.

(C) Childhood history.

(D) Relationships and marriage history.

(86) A psychiatric mental health nurse practitioner can use the following to get information about the current mental state of the patient:

(A) Adverse childhood experiences score.

(B) Physical examination.

(C) Mental status examination.

(D) Psychiatric history.

(87) The general description of the patient is included in the intake section about:

(A) Perceptual disturbances.

(B) Motor activity.

(C) Speech.

(D) Appearance and behavior.

(88) A patient in a manic episode has:

(A) Pressured speech.

(B) Decreased amount of speech.

(C) Timid speech.

(D) Slow speech.

(89) A 43-year-old patient talks about the death of her husband. She reports feeling very depressed and unable to get out of bed, but during the interview, she laughs hysterically. The psychiatric mental health nurse practitioner writes that the woman's affect and mood are:

(A) Incongruent, depressed.

(B) Congruent, euphoric.

(C) Incongruent, euphoric.

(D) Congruent, depressed.

(90) Which word can be used to describe a normal thought process?

(A) Goal-directed.

(B) Tangential.

(C) Circumstantial.

(D) Perseveration.

(91) Which of the following is not a perceptual disturbance?

(A) Illusion.

(B) Hallucination.

(C) Depersonalization.

(D) Delusion.

(92) A psychiatric mental health nurse wants to test the patient's alertness, orientation, and concentration. In what intake section do these elements belong?

(A) Thought form.

(B) Thought process.

(C) Cognition.

(D) Speech.

(93) The patient's understanding of the presence of his psychiatric illness is called:

(A) Judgment.

(B) Insight.

(C) Cognition.

(D) Perception.

(94) What is the strongest risk factor for suicide?

(A) Previous suicide attempts.

(B) Lack of insight.

(C) The presence of hallucinations.

(D) Family history of suicide attempts.

(95) A patient is fixated on a car accident he saw in the news earlier in the day. The psychiatric mental health nurse practitioner attempts to change the topic multiple times. The patient repeatedly goes back to that topic. What is the patient's thought process called?

(A) Flight of ideas.

(B) Loose associations.

(C) Perseveration.

(D) Clang associations.

(96) To assess suicide risk, the psychiatric mental health nurse practitioner can:

(A) Ask the patient openly if they have suicidal thoughts.

(B) Look through the patient's medical history.

(C) Order a complete blood count.

(D) Observe the patient's behavior.

(97) During the interview, a psychiatric mental health nurse practitioner asks a suicidal patient: "What is the main reason you have not gone further with your plan of suicide?" The patient reports that the main reason he is still alive is that he does not want to harm his brother. The psychiatric mental health nurse practitioner:

(A) Ignores this information since it is not relevant to suicide risk.

(B) Orders an EEG.

(C) Asks the patient if he hears voices.

(D) Treats this information as important since it is relevant to the patient's suicide risk.

(98) Which of the following areas is not included in the risk assessment?

(A) Risk of self-harm.

(B) Likelihood of substance abuse.

(C) Family history of psychiatric disorders.

(D) Risk of self-neglect.

(99) A female 32-year-old patient with a history of 10 years of intravenous drug use complains of a depressed mood and lack of interest in activities that used to bring her pleasure. Other than the psychiatric interview and physical examination, which test should the psychiatric mental health nurse order?

(A) MRI.

(B) EEG.

(C) CT.

(D) Hepatitis C test.

(100) What is the healthcare model that is focused on making patients feel involved in their treatment and care journey?

(A) Doctor-centered care.

(B) Symptom-centered care.

(C) Disease-centered care.

(D) Client-centered care.

(101) A psychiatric mental health nurse practitioner who is educated in client-centered care can:

(A) Manage the patient's symptoms.

(B) Use a holistic approach and consider the well-being of the patient as a whole instead of isolating the illness.

(C) Communicate only with the family about the patient and include them in the treatment plan.

(D) Focus on the creation of an appropriate pharmacologic treatment plan.

(102) A patient who is in a state of psychosis is taken to the psychiatric emergency department. The environment in which the patient is examined:

(A) Will not influence the patient's cooperation.

(B) Is irrelevant for the initial interaction.

(C) Must be clean—nothing else matters.

(D) Should be welcoming and safe.

(103) What is an element of client-centered care?

(A) Respect for the patients' preferences, needs, and values.

(B) Cognitive-behavioral therapy.

(C) Eye movement desensitization and reprocessing (EMDR)

(D) A form the patient signs, agreeing to voluntary hospitalization.

(104) Which statement below is true about coordination and integration of care?

(A) Transitions between different providers in different phases of treatment should be smooth and not cause confusion and stress.

(B) The psychiatric mental health nurse practitioner is not responsible for the provision of formal and informal services.

(C) The patient can be easily transitioned between many types of providers.

(D) The coordination and integration of care does not influence recovery.

(105) A 25-year-old female patient is diagnosed with schizophrenia. She complains of worry about how the diagnosis will impact her career. According to the principles of client-centered care, the psychiatric mental health nurse practitioner should:

(A) Inform the patient of the most appropriate career choices for someone with schizophrenia.

(B) Talk to the doctor about the patient's worries and suggest that he increase the dose of benzodiazepines.

(C) Dismiss the patient's worries and tell her that she should think about them in the future once her condition is stable.

(D) Show empathy and reassure the patient.

(106) Which of the following statements does not follow the principles of client-centered care?

(A) The psychiatric mental health nurse practitioner should empower the patient's family and friends and inform them that they can have a positive impact on the health of their loved one.

(B) The psychiatric mental health nurse practitioner should be aware of the impact of the sociocultural background of the patient on the healthcare journey.

(C) Trust is necessary for a productive relationship between the healthcare provider and the patient.

(D) The patient should not have any responsibilities in the treatment journey.

(107) What is not a principle of client-centered care?

(A) Psychopharmacology treatment plan.

(B) Involvement of family and friends.

(C) Clear information, education, and support.

(D) Coordination and integration of care.

(108) A 37-year-old male patient is put on long-acting injectable paliperidone palmitate treatment. On a follow-up visit, laboratory results show increased prolactin levels. According to the principles of client-centered care, the psychiatric mental health nurse practitioner should:

(A) Inform the patient of the increased prolactin levels.

(B) Order an MRI of the brain to check for a tumor of the pituitary gland.

(C) Ignore the finding since it is a common side effect of this medication.

(D) Stop the treatment with paliperidone palmitate.

(109) Which of the following best exemplifies the principles of client-centered care for mental health nursing?

(A) The nurse creates a treatment plan without input from the client to ensure it is medically sound.

(B) The nurse encourages the client to participate in decisions about their care and respects their preferences and values.

(C) The nurse prioritizes medication compliance over understanding the client's personal experiences.

(D) The nurse minimizes family involvement to maintain client confidentiality.

(110) Peter is a 34-year-old lawyer. He complains of anxiety, nervousness, and insomnia. During the interview, he reports that he abuses substances, but he is hesitant to share the type, amount, and route of use. He is afraid that his friends might find out about his habit. What should the psychiatric mental health nurse practitioner do in this situation?

(A) Inform the patient that the information shared during the interview is confidential.

(B) Inform the patient that his family must know about his substance use.

(C) Order a toxicology screening test without the patient's knowledge.

(D) Accept the patient's wish not to disclose the information.

(111) John is a 45-year-old patient who has two teenage sons. He complains of auditory hallucinations. His mood is depressed. He is hesitant to seek help because he thinks that might negatively influence his son's reputation. "School is cruel, and when a kid has a crazy dad, that makes it even crueler," he says. What should the psychiatric mental health nurse practitioner do in this situation?

(A) Ignore the patient's worries and insist that he take the medication.

(B) Talk to the school principal about John's situation.

(C) Be empathetic toward John and provide comfort and reassurance. Explain that the benefits of treatment outweigh the cons.

(D) Talk to the patient's sons about John's worries.

(112) Which of the following statements is false about client-centered care in psychiatry?

(A) Psychiatry used to be criticized because it categorized individuals into mental illnesses and didn't pay attention to their different backgrounds, such as culture, religion, past trauma, and personal experiences.

(B) Healthcare providers in psychiatry are often required to restrict the individual freedoms of patients to achieve the best clinical outcome.

(C) Most individuals feel as if they are completely involved in their mental health treatment.

(D) The curriculum for trainees in psychiatry medicine does not include client-centered care.

(113) In order for psychiatric mental health providers to balance respect for patients' human rights and providing the best care, they must be aware of:

(A) The DSM-V.

(B) Human rights and relevant legislation.

(C) The second amendment.

(D) The patient's previous medical history.

(114) When a management plan is developed in collaboration with the patient, sometimes the psychiatric mental health nurse practitioner:

(A) Can dismiss patient's preferences if they're not relevant to current guidelines.

(B) Might have to consult other doctors if the patient insists on a certain type of therapy.

(C) Will have to give up on a patient if he has unrealistic expectations of the treatment.

(D) Might have to choose a treatment that is not the best according to current evidence-based medicine.

(115) When it comes to the well-being of doctors and nurses, client-centered care:

(A) Ignores medical professionals' health.

(B) Puts patient needs above the well-being of healthcare providers.

(C) Does not recognize healthcare providers' needs.

(D) Aims to improve work satisfaction and reduce burnout levels.

(116) Which of the following is false about client-centered care?

(A) Client-centered care and the goals of personal recovery both draw attention to the patient's recovery goals.

(B) The client-centered care approach aims to improve the lives of healthcare providers.

(C) Client-centered care emphasizes guidelines and protocols.

(D) Patients should always be treated with dignity, and the doctor should listen to what they have to say and consider their input.

(117) Which of the following is most important to consider when providing patient education?

(A) The patient's literacy level and preferred learning style.

(B) The nurse's own expertise and knowledge.

(C) The availability of online educational resources.

(D) The use of medical jargon to ensure accuracy.

(118) The process of learning can be impacted by factors such as the meaningfulness of the material, retention of learning, transfer or learning, and other individual factors. Which primary individual factor is defined as the capacity of the individual to learn and use new information?

(A) Education level.

(B) Talent.

(C) Knowledge.

(D) Intelligence.

(119) Learning has a hierarchical nature. This means that:

(A) Some material is more important than others.

(B) Some people are allowed to learn certain material, and some are not, based on their intelligence level.

(C) New knowledge is built upon previous knowledge, and new and old knowledge are connected.

(D) There is no connection between learning materials.

(120) Which characteristics will contribute to a patient learning new and complex material more easily?

(A) The location of their home.

(B) A bachelor's degree in organic chemistry.

(C) The number of siblings they have.

(D) Their father's level of education.

(121) How does anxiety influence the process of learning?

(A) Anxiety increases creativity and makes learning creative concepts easier.

(B) Anxiety has no impact on the learning process.

(C) Anxiety increases a person's ability to learn.

(D) Anxiety creates hopelessness, which can make the person unwilling to learn new material.

(122) What is not a method that can maximize the effectiveness of learning?

(A) Whole versus part.

(B) Active participation.

(C) Distribution of practice.

(D) Passivity and resistance.

(123) When a patient exhibits active participation, he:

(A) Asks questions and make comments.

(B) Talks to other patients.

(C) Zones out during a conversation.

(D) Refuses to read educational material.

(124) Which of the following is false about the optimization of learning?

(A) How you present the material is an important factor in the learning process.

(B) Active participation increases individuals' ability to learn both cognitive and psychomotor tasks.

(C) In order to achieve optimal learning of a skill, practice time needs to be long enough and organized in a way that enables continuity between response and reinforcement.

(D) People learn better when they pay attention only to discrete parts, not the entirety of the material.

(125) Which of the following statements is false about the process of learning?

(A) Distribution of practice can be achieved through frequent practice sessions, sequencing tasks, and an emphasis on speed over accuracy.

(B) There is no need to inform people about their test results since that might discourage them.

(C) Even though there are variations in people's abilities and motivations to learn, certain methods can maximize the effectiveness and efficiency of learning for the majority of people.

(D) Break down a task into smaller manageable units to make it easier for learners to focus and avoid feelings of overwhelm.

(126) How does the meaningfulness of material facilitate the learning process?

(A) It increases the motivation of the learner.

(B) It increases the cognitive capacity of the learner.

(C) It increases the intelligence of the learner.

(D) It reduces the anxiety of the learner.

(127) What kind of transfer of learning occurs when the individual uses old concepts to understand or learn concepts with increased complexity?

(A) Identical transfer.

(B) Heterogenous transfer.

(C) Vertical transfer.

(D) Horizontal transfer.

(128) A 30-year-old male patient who has used heroin for the past eight years expresses a wish to cure his addiction. The patient is starting to consider change, but he is still not ready to take action, which means that he is in:

(A) The first (pre-contemplative) stage of change.

(B) The second (contemplative) stage of change.

(C) The third (action) stage of change.

(D) The fourth (maintenance) stage of change.

(129) A 34-year-old female patient who abuses amphetamines is very irritable. She frequently fights with her husband, and she has problems with her coworkers. Her family wants her to stop her substance abuse, but she insists that she does not have a problem. Psychoeducation should help:

(A) Teach the patient better coping mechanisms.

(B) Teach the patient better behavioral actions.

(C) Teach the patient how to prevent relapse.

(D) Teach the patient about how addiction affects her life.

(130) To assess patients' learning style:

(A) Ask if they prefer to learn during the day or the night.

(B) Ask what medications they are using.

(C) Ask if they enjoyed their elementary school years.

(D) Ask about their ACE score.

(131) Which of the following is false about learning objectives?

(A) Learning objectives are short term.

(B) Learning objectives are long term.

(C) Learning objectives are measurable.

(D) Learning objectives are attainable.

(132) Which of the following is not used in the assessment of a patient's learning style?

(A) Checklists and questionnaires.

(B) List of prescribed medication.

(C) Information from the family.

(D) Information from other healthcare staff.

(133) The first part of the patient education process is to:

(A) Assess the patient's learning needs.

(B) Assess the patient's learning style.

(C) Assess the patient's readiness to learn.

(D) Develop learning objectives.

(134) When they develop goals for psychoeducation, clinicians should consider the patient's:

(A) Readiness to learn.

(B) Socioeconomic status.

(C) Medical comorbidities.

(D) Personality type.

(135) Retroactive inhibition occurs when:

(A) Previous knowledge interferes with learning new material.

(B) Learning material gradually fades away.

(C) New material interferes with the retrieval of old material.

(D) The material has no meaning.

(136) Which of the following does not have any influence on content retention?

(A) The meaning of the material.

(B) How much the learner uses the material after learning it.

(C) The educator's intelligence level.

(D) Traumatic and intervening situations.

(137) Shared patterns of belief, knowledge, and feelings that influence people's behavior are called:

(A) Ethnicity.

(B) Gender identity.

(C) Culture.

(D) Religious belief.

(138) The assumption that people from the same cultural or ethnic groups all exhibit the same behavior is called:

(A) Stereotyping.

(B) Archetyping.

(C) Categorization.

(D) Classification.

(139) A type of practice that minimizes misunderstandings that may arise between healthcare providers and patients because of cultural diversity is called:

(A) Trauma-informed care.

(B) Person-centered care.

(C) Client-centered care.

(D) Culturally competent care.

(140) Which of the following statements is false about cultural competence when caring for patients who are members of the LGBTQ community?

(A) To provide culturally competent care for LGBTQ individuals, healthcare workers should avoid discrimination, stigmatization, and unconscious biases and aim for equality of care.

(B) LGBTQ community members are faced with many challenges throughout their lives.

(C) To provide culturally competent care, healthcare providers should know the common terms used by the LGBTQ community.

(D) Healthcare providers are allowed to use slang if the patient chooses to use it.

(141) Androgyny is defined as:

(A) A person who is attracted to both females and males.

(B) The individual's sense of gender, which may be different from the assigned sex at birth.

(C) A person who is in between genders and has both male and female characteristics.

(D) A person who is attracted to members of the opposite sex.

(142) The appearance, social behavior, style, or mannerisms associated with masculinity or femininity are known as:

(A) Transphobia.

(B) Gender identity.

(C) Gender expression.

(D) Gender neutrality.

(143) What is not a challenge that healthcare providers have when caring for LGBTQ patients?

(A) Difficulties openly discussing sexual health-related problems, along with a lack of familiarity with gender modification surgery.

(B) Patients' reluctance to share sexual practices.

(C) Forgetting to use gender-neutral terms (e.g., significant other, partner).

(D) Previous positive experiences with clinicians.

(144) Which of the following statements about members of the LGBTQ community is false?

(A) Lesbian women, gay men, and bisexual people have a higher chance of suffering from depression.

(B) Lesbian women, gay men, and bisexual people have a higher chance of suffering from substance abuse.

(C) Lesbian women, gay men, and bisexual people have a lower chance of dying by suicide.

(D) Lesbian women, gay men, and bisexual people experience minority stress.

(145) Which of the following tools is commonly used to screen for alcohol use disorders?

(A) MMSE.

(B) HAM-D.

(C) CAGE.

(D) PANSS.

(146) During conversations, Native American people may appear:

(A) Very aggressive and confrontational.

(B) Reserved and silent.

(C) Loud and talkative.

(D) Expressive and emotional.

(147) What is a healer called in some Native American cultures?

(A) The old lady.

(B) Granny.

(C) Doctor.

(D) Shaman.

(148) What is a significant issue in some Native American cultures?

(A) Addiction to alcohol.

(B) Addiction to pornography.

(C) Addiction to gambling.

(D)Addiction to heroin.

(149) According to Erik Erikson's stages of psychosocial development, which developmental challenge is a 45-year-old individual most likely to face?

(A) Trust vs. Mistrust.

(B) Initiative vs. Guilt.

(C) Generativity vs. Stagnation.

(D) Integrity vs. Despair.

(150) Which of the following statements is correct about Asian American culture?

(A) Some Asian Americans consider lack of eye contact disrespectful.

(B) Some Asian Americans often raise their voices in communication.

(C) Some Asian Americans prefer eccentric behavior.

(D) Some Asian Americans consider eye contact disrespectful.

Test 1: Answers and Explanations

(1) (B) The development of a healthy personality.

Erikson's theory of psychosocial development consists of eight stages of ego development that are characterized by psychosocial crises (basic conflicts) that reflect the needs of the individual and conflict with the needs of society. The resolution of a crisis can cause the development of a healthy personality or psychosocial regression. A healthy personality can be developed with the successful resolution of the crisis in each stage. An individual who successfully completes the stage acquires basic virtues that can be used to resolve the next crises.

(2) (A) Trust versus mistrust.

In the first stage of psychosocial development, the basic conflict is trust versus mistrust. In this stage, the infant is completely dependent on primary caregivers. Therefore, it looks up to them for the fulfillment of its basic needs, security, and stability. The infant learns about the world and society through interactions with its parents. The task during this stage is for the infant to learn whether other people can be relied upon for the fulfillment of the infant's basic needs.

(3) (D) The infant does not trust the world.

During the first stage of psychosocial development, if the parents fail to provide security, comfort, care, and affection, the infant will develop mistrust. The infant will learn that the world is inconsistent, unreliable, and unpredictable. If the parents successfully provide the infant with security, comfort, affection, food, and warmth, the infant will develop a sense of trust in the world and learn that others can be dependable.

(4) (C) Second stage of psychosocial development.

In the second stage of psychosocial development, the major crisis is autonomy versus shame and doubt. During this stage, children start to develop more autonomy and a sense of independence, which is manifested in increased mobility and the discovery of new abilities, such as how to dress, pick up toys, and others. Children in this stage start to explore the world and their interests.

(5) (A) If parents successfully encourage their children's independence, then the children will develop self-confidence and autonomy.

During the second stage of psychosocial development, parents serve as a secure base from which toddlers can explore their newly found autonomy. Children then feel comfortable to explore the external environment and freely make choices. If the parents are too controlling and overly critical, children will develop shame and doubt in their own competence.

(6) (D) Third stage of psychosocial development.

The third stage of psychosocial development is also called the locomotor stage. Children start to become active and master their environment. They learn basic skills such as how to count, speak, plan etc. They start to understand that actions have a purpose. The basic conflict during this stage is initiative versus guilt.

(7) (B) It might cause guilt, which can damage the child's curiosity and creativity.

The four-year-old is in the third stage of psychosocial development, also called the locomotor stage. During this stage, children may start to ask a lot of questions since their curiosity about the world starts to grow. When parents respond to a child's question with annoyance, the child might develop guilt. This damages the child's curiosity and creativity.

(8) (B) Fourth stage of psychosocial development.

The fourth stage of psychosocial development is industry versus inferiority. During this stage, children start elementary school. They have interactions with their peers and teachers. Children are expected to learn new skills and develop their individuality and moral code. Teachers and parents have increased expectations, and children start to develop their confidence based on their abilities to fulfill those expectations.

(9) (D) The basic conflict in this stage is initiative versus guilt.

This is false. The basic conflict of the fourth stage of psychosocial development is industry versus inferiority. If children are encouraged and praised for their accomplishments and abilities, they will develop industry. Children become responsible, complete tasks, and put in effort while delaying pleasure. If children are criticized, they may feel incapable and develop inferiority.

(10) (C) Fifth stage of psychosocial development.

The fifth stage of psychosocial development is the transition from childhood to adulthood. In this stage, adolescents explore their identity and their role in the world. The basic conflict is about identity versus role confusion, and the main existential question is: "Who am I, and what can I be?" Adolescents become concerned with how they appear to other people. They become curious about occupational, political, gender, religious, and sexual identities.

(11) (B) Implementing a strict bedtime routine.

Establishing a consistent routine helps regulate the body's internal clock (circadian rhythm) and promotes better sleep hygiene. By going to bed and waking up at the same time every day, patients can train their bodies to recognize when it is time to sleep, which can lead to improved sleep onset and quality.

(12) (A) A normal occurrence.

It is normal to experience role confusion during the fifth stage of psychosocial development. Adolescents may become confused about their role in the world, and they will experiment with different activities in order to sort out that confusion. According to Erikson, adolescents go through an identity crisis. The successful resolution of an identity crisis leads to the development of an integrated sense of self.

(13) (A) Parents should allow their children to develop their own identity.

It is necessary for parents to allow children to develop their own identity. Forcing them into a chosen identity (a cardiologist) may cause rebellious behavior and a negative view of self. For the successful resolution of the fifth psychosocial stage of development, the daughter needs to be given enough space and time so she can freely explore who she truly is.

(14) (C) Unresolved identity issues leave a person confused about their direction in life and role in society.

This is the stage in which the transition from childhood to adulthood occurs. In this stage, adolescents explore their identity and their role in the world. If adolescents leave this stage with unresolved identity issues, they will become confused about their direction in life and their role in society. Consequently, they may develop a weak sense of self. An individual who successfully resolves this stage develops a strong identity and consistent values.

(15) (C) Intimacy vs. Isolation.

The sixth stage of Erik Erikson's psychological development is Intimacy vs. Isolation. This stage occurs during young adulthood, where individuals focus on forming intimate, loving relationships with others. Successful completion of this stage leads to strong relationships, while failure results in loneliness and isolation.

(16) (C) Consider what they have left behind for their community.

During the seventh stage of psychosocial development, adults aim to achieve generativity through contributions to the world and society. Since people in this stage are closer to the end of their lives, their main concern is what they have left behind for the community. Generativity is achieved when adults make an effort to contribute to positive societal changes that improve the lives of future generations.

(17) (D) Adults who don't achieve generativity feel connected to their community.

This is false. Generativity is achieved when adults make an effort to contribute to positive societal changes that improve the lives of future generations. If a person has failed to work toward a meaningful goal in life, they will feel stagnation and emptiness. Adults who have failed to achieve the virtue of care might feel a great disconnection with society and their community.

(18) (D) Create and maintain a comfortable home.

Tasks that middle adults engage in include the creation of and maintenance of a comfortable home, creative use of leisure time, the expression of love in various ways, etc. Parenthood is another significant task during this part of life. When they teach values to children, adults gain a great sense of generativity.

(19) (A) People retire and have more time to reflect on their lives.

The eighth stage is the last of Erikson's stages of psychosocial development. In this stage, people reflect on the meaning of their lives. As they retire, productivity decreases, and they have more time for activities that do not involve work.

(20) (D) Ego integrity versus despair.

People who feel like they have achieved their goals and found a sense of purpose will develop ego integrity. Individuals who develop ego integrity can look back on their lives and see them as successful and productive. Individuals who are unsatisfied with their lives, who feel as if they have been unproductive or empty, will develop despair. They might become depressed and fearful of death.

(21) (B) Thyroid function tests.

This patient's depressive mood might be due to thyroid dysfunction, which can be suspected because of the physical examination (dry skin, intolerance to cold temperatures). Hypothyroidism is a common cause of psychiatric symptoms such as depression, cognitive impairment, memory loss, irritability, and myxedema coma. Patients who present with depressive symptoms and cognitive impairment should be screened for hypothyroidism since the psychiatric symptoms are reversible if the underlying cause is treated.

(22) (C) Graves's disease.

Increased anxiety and panic attacks that co-occur with palpitations, excessive sweating, and weight loss may be a sign of hyperthyroidism. Hyperthyroidism is caused by Graves's disease, toxic multinodular goiter, toxic adenoma, postpartum hyperthyroidism, and a factitious hyperthyroid state. Hyperthyroidism presents with irritability, diaphoresis, palpitations, weight loss, dyspnea, tachycardia, excessive sweating, and fatigue. The most common psychiatric symptoms associated with hyperthyroidism are depression, anxiety, and cognitive impairment.

(23) (B) Cushing's syndrome.

Cushing's syndrome most commonly occurs when there is increased secretion of cortisol by the adrenal gland or excessive exogenous glucocorticoid administration (e.g., in the treatment of chronic inflammatory diseases). Other causes of Cushing's syndrome include endogenous overproduction of glucocorticoid (e.g., a glucocorticoid-secreting tumor) or diseases of the pituitary gland. Cushing's syndrome presents with somatic and psychiatric symptoms. Psychiatric symptoms of Cushing's syndrome resolve when the hypercortisolemia is normalized.

(24) (D) Serum cortisol and ACTH measurement.

This patient might have adrenal insufficiency. Therefore, the psychiatric mental health nurse practitioner should order serum adrenocorticotropic hormone (ACTH) and cortisol tests. Adrenal insufficiency causes nonspecific symptoms that may overlap with other psychiatric diseases. Therefore, these patients are often misdiagnosed with major depressive disorder, dementia, or somatoform disorders. Psychiatric symptoms resolve once the hormone deficiency is corrected.

(25) (A) Vitamin B1 deficiency.

Vitamin B1 (thiamine) deficiency causes Wernicke-Korsakoff syndrome. Wernicke encephalopathy is a syndrome characterized by a triad of ataxia, cognitive deficiencies in attention and orientation, and oculomotor dysfunction. Korsakoff syndrome consists of anterograde and retrograde memory loss. Long-term memory is preserved in patients with Korsakoff syndrome. The diagnosis is confirmed with laboratory measurements of serum thiamine.

(26) (B) Orders serum vitamin B12 tests.

This patient's clinical presentation and surgical history may indicate a vitamin B12 deficiency. Vitamin B12 deficiency occurs due to malabsorption, such as in pernicious anemia or gastric/small bowel resection. Vitamin B12 deficiency is associated with many neuropsychiatric symptoms like depression, anxiety/panic disorder, hallucinations, delusions, insomnia, mania, psychosis, sensory polyneuropathy (impaired sense of vibration and proprioception), dysgeusia, urinary/fecal incontinence, cerebellar ataxia, cognitive impairment, spasticity, obtundation, and decreased visual acuity.

(27) (D) Hypocalcemia is not associated with psychiatric symptoms.

This is false. Neuropsychiatric symptoms can occur as a result of elevated or decreased calcium levels in the blood. Hypocalcemia causes seizures, disorientation, confusion, emotional lability, delirium, anxiety, depression, and psychosis. Correction of the hypocalcemia with vitamin D and calcium supplementation will resolve the neuropsychiatric symptoms. Hypercalcemia causes confusion, weakness, lethargy, drowsiness, and depressive symptoms. Severe hypercalcemia may cause psychosis, stupor, coma, or death.

(28) (D) Lithium.

Hypercalcemia may occur as a result of lithium therapy. Primary hyperparathyroidism and malignancy are the most common causes of hypercalcemia. Severe hypercalcemia may cause psychosis, stupor, coma, or death.

(29) (A) Wilson's disease.

Wilson's disease, also called hepatolenticular degeneration, is an autosomal recessive disorder that affects the hepatic transport of copper. This defect causes excessive copper deposition in organs, especially in the liver and the brain. Excessive copper deposition is responsible for organ injury. Wilson's disease causes both neurologic and psychiatric symptoms. Neurologic symptoms include choreoathetosis, tremors, dystonia, ataxia, and cognitive impairment. Psychiatric symptoms include irritability, disinhibition, depression, aggression, and recklessness.

(30) (B) Order 24-hour urine copper quantification.

The presence of the Kayser-Fleischer ring is suggestive of Wilson's disease, also called hepatolenticular degeneration. The diagnosis can be made with 24-hour urine copper quantification. Proper diagnosis and treatment can enable these individuals to have a normal life and prevent the onset of neuropsychiatric symptoms.

(31) (C) Systemic lupus erythematosus.

SLE is an autoimmune disorder caused by the presence of autoantibodies that damage several organs. The organs most commonly affected are the skin, kidneys, lungs, and central nervous system. Symptoms of SLE include fatigue, fever, arthralgias, myalgias, weight loss, butterfly rash, photosensitivity, mucous ulcers, and Raynaud's phenomenon. Neuropsychiatric symptoms occur due to the presence of autoantibodies directed against neuronal membranes and antibodies against NMDA receptors (N-methyl-D-aspartate).

(32) (D) The patient might have developed psychosis either because of his disease or because of treatment with corticosteroids.

Psychiatric manifestations of SLE include depression, mood disorders, anxiety disorders, psychosis, and cognitive decline (memory impairment, learning difficulties). Treatment consists of corticosteroids and immunosuppressive medications like azathioprine and cyclophosphamide. In certain cases, steroid treatment induces psychiatric symptoms. It is difficult to differentiate steroid psychosis from psychosis caused by CNS lupus, and such a diagnosis requires close collaboration between psychiatrists and rheumatologists. Lupus psychosis is treated with antipsychotics.

(33) (C) Generalized anxiety disorder.

Patients with esophageal dysmotility most commonly suffer from major depressive disorder (up to 52%), generalized anxiety disorder (36%), somatization disorder (20%), and substance-use disorders (20%). Esophageal dysmotility is a cause of non-cardiac chest pain that leads many patients to seek psychiatric consultation.

(34) (D) The most common psychiatric disorders found in patients with irritable bowel syndrome are schizophrenia, schizoaffective disorder, and OCD.

Psychiatric disorders are frequently found in patients who suffer from IBS. The most common ones are panic disorder (26%), social phobia (26%), generalized anxiety disorder (26%), and major depressive disorder (23%). Irritable bowel syndrome is associated with stress due to increased sensitivity of the enteric nervous system to stress. Emotional stress causes increased sympathetic nervous system activity, which causes inhibition of gastric motility.

(35) (D) Tricyclic antidepressants.

Tricyclic antidepressants are beneficial for patients who suffer from diarrhea and IBS due to their anticholinergic effect. Most patients with IBS improve with low-dose antidepressants or antianxiety medications, even if they don't have a psychiatric disorder.

(36) (A) Diazepam.

Increased carbon dioxide levels in the blood can cause panic attacks in patients with COPD. Benzodiazepines are not useful for panic attacks in such patients because they suppress respiratory function. Neuroleptics may be given to patients with COPD to manage fear and panic.

(37) (A) Anxiety disorder.

Anxiety is the most common psychiatric disorder in patients with gastroesophageal reflux disease. Gastroesophageal reflux and peptic ulcer disease cause epigastric non-cardiac chest pain one to three hours after a meal. Major risk factors of peptic ulcer disease are infection with *Helicobacter Pylori* and excessive use of nonsteroidal anti-inflammatory drugs. Many patients who have non-ulcer dyspepsia suffer from a psychiatric comorbidity.

(38) (C) Psychiatric symptoms seen in patients with COPD may be due to chronic hypoxia or treatment with corticosteroid medications.

Chronic hypoxia in COPD causes cognitive deficits and mood disorders. Patients may present with depression, mood lability, or delirium. Increased carbon dioxide levels in the blood can cause panic attacks.

(39) (D) Obstructive sleep apnea.

Patients who report chronic fatigue, excessive daytime sleepiness, depression, poor motivation, and impaired concentration should be screened for sleep apnea during the psychiatric interview. OSA can be defined as an obstruction of the upper airways that causes complete cessation of airflow during sleep. The obstructive episodes usually last for 10 seconds or more, and they occur most commonly during REM sleep.

(40) (B) Cardiac morbidity or mortality.

A type A personality increases the risk of myocardial infarction. People with type A personalities are ambitious, competitive, impatient, aggressive, alert, have a high potential for anger, get easily irritated, and suffer from muscle tension. They can describe themselves as workaholics, and they pride themselves in being resistant to emotional "weakness." These patients feel the need to control their bodies.

(41) (D) Women tend to have more negative symptoms compared to men.

This is false. Women do not have more negative symptoms of schizophrenia compared to men. Women tend to have more dysphoria, paranoid delusions, and hallucinations compared to men. Men usually have an earlier onset of the disease, more negative symptoms, and a poorer prognosis. Men are more affected by schizophrenia than women.

(42) (B) Auditory hallucinations.

Auditory hallucinations are most common in schizophrenia. However, all five senses may be affected. Tactile, gustatory, and olfactory hallucinations are very rare, and their presence may point toward an underlying neurological or medical cause of psychosis.

Patients hear voices that can be insulting or threatening. The voices may talk to each other.

(43) (B) Psychosis.

This patient probably has a psychotic disorder. Signs that point toward the diagnosis: he has religious and grandiose delusions (he thinks he is the messiah, come to save the world). He may have auditory hallucinations since he talks to himself. His speech is disorganized ("word salad"), and he is agitated. All these symptoms occur in the presentation of a psychotic episode.

(44) (D) The hallmark of schizophrenia is an elevated, expansive, grandiose mood.

This is false. An elevated, expansive, grandiose mood is the hallmark of a manic episode seen in bipolar disorder, not schizophrenia. Affective symptoms of schizophrenia may range from anhedonia to extreme rage, depression, and anxiety. Patients often have a flat or blunted affect. Behavior is unusual, and it may range from silliness to unpredictable anger.

(45) (A) Hallucinations, delusions, and disorganized, bizarre behaviors.

Positive symptoms of schizophrenia include hallucinations, delusions, and disorganized, bizarre behaviors. Delusions can be persecutory, grandiose, erotomanic, jealous, religious, and somatic. Patients may believe they are being controlled by an outside entity or that they can control the outside world. Hallucinations are most commonly auditory, but all five senses may be affected. The voices patients hear may insult or threaten them. The voices may also talk to each other.

(46) (B) Manic episode.

This patient's clinical presentation is consistent with a manic episode. The hallmark of a manic episode is an increased, uninhibited, or irritable mood that lasts for at least a week. The patient in a manic episode is very talkative, amusing, euphoric, and speaks with a sense of urgency, which is referred to as pressured speech. The patient may exhibit unusual risky behaviors such as unrestrained shopping sprees, unsafe promiscuous behavior, and excessive substance use. Patients have a decreased need for sleep and are hyperactive.

(47) (C) Major depressive disorder.

This patient's clinical presentation is consistent with major depressive disorder. The clinical presentation of a major depressive disorder consists of a loss of pleasure (anhedonia), a decrease or increase in weight or appetite, sleep, or activity, a decrease in energy, psychomotor retardation, dysphoria, impaired concentration, depressive thoughts filled with worthlessness and guilt, and suicidal ideation. To diagnose major depressive disorder, the symptoms must be present for at least one week.

(48) (B) Dysthymia.

Dysthymic disorder is a less severe form of major depressive disorder. The hallmark of dysthymia is a continuous depressive mood that begins in childhood or adolescence.

(49) (A) Neurocognitive disorders are caused by a medical or neurological condition that manifests as psychiatric and/or neurologic symptomatology and changes in cognition.

Cognitive disorders are characterized by a disruption in one or two of the following domains: language, memory, judgment, orientation, interpersonal relationships, problem-solving, and praxis (performing functions). They are often accompanied by abnormal behavior. The deficit in cognition is a major change from the patient's previous level of functioning. These disorders most commonly affect older adults, but they may occur at any age. Delirium and dementia are the most common neurocognitive disorders.

(50) (B) Delirium.

Delirium is a syndrome with an acute onset characterized by a short-term decline in consciousness and cognition. Delirium may occur due to a general medical condition, substance use, multiple physical health etiologies, and others (e.g., sleep deprivation, medications, etc.). Older adults are most affected by delirium. The disturbance of consciousness usually develops over hours to a few days, and it fluctuates during the day.

(51) (A) Dementia.

Dementia is characterized by a progressive decline of cognitive abilities in the setting of a clear consciousness. The decline causes major impairment in the patient's occupational and social functioning.

(52) (A) Paranoid personality disorder.

Patients with paranoid personality disorders are excessively suspicious of others. They are distrustful and may interpret other's intentions as threatening, deceptive, or hostile. They frequently have trouble with interpersonal relationships due to pathological jealousy.

(53) (B) Schizotypal personality disorder.

This patient most likely has schizotypal personality disorder. Patients with this personality disorder often have superstitious beliefs and may believe they possess special powers. The hallmark of schizotypal personality disorder is difficulty in the maintenance of interpersonal relationships and eccentric behavior. These patients have disturbed thought and communication with the absence of the actual thought disorder. They are at risk of developing psychotic symptoms when they are under stress.

(54) (C) Antisocial personality disorder.

Antisocial personality disorder is characterized by a pervasive disrespect for other people's rights. These patients are frequently diagnosed with conduct disorder in their childhood or have evidence of behaviors that point towards conduct disorder. At first, these patients may appear charming or manipulative. They may lie, abuse others, or commit crimes. They have no remorse for their actions and act as if they have no conscience.

(55) (A) Patients with BPD have an intense fear of abandonment.

An intense fear of abandonment is the hallmark of borderline personality disorder. Borderline personality disorder is characterized by chaotic interpersonal relationships, intense fear of abandonment and frantic efforts to avoid it, impulsive behavior, affective instability, chronic sense of emptiness, identity disturbance, black-and-white thinking (often called splitting), chronic or recurrent suicidality, and dissociative symptoms.

(56) (D) Narcissistic personality disorder.

The hallmark of narcissistic personality disorder is an exaggerated sense of self-importance and grandiosity. These patients lack empathy for others and may exhibit exploitative behaviors and arrogance. They may expect special treatment and validation from others.

(57) (D) Schizotypal personality disorder.

Schizotypal personality disorder is not a part of cluster C (anxious) personality disorders. Cluster C includes avoidant, dependent, and obsessive-compulsive personality disorders. Patients with avoidant personality disorder lack confidence and are very sensitive to rejection. Patients with a dependent personality disorder are submissive and dependent on others. Obsessive-compulsive personality disorder is characterized by a preoccupation with order, rules, and regulations.

(58) (B) Ruminations about potential dangers.

Patients with anxiety catastrophize and ruminate on potential dangers. Their thoughts are rapid, disorganized, and negative. Patients who have panic attacks may think they are dying or having a heart attack.

(59) (C) Agoraphobia.

Agoraphobia is a type of anxiety disorder characterized by a fear of situations or places that might be difficult to escape. It causes occupational and social dysfunction since patients with agoraphobia may find it very difficult to leave their homes. It may occur with or without a panic disorder.

(60) (C) Coping styles.

When a person endures a stressful situation, the set of behaviors they use to deal with the stress is called a coping style. One way of coping is to consciously seek support from others. Another way is through conscious cognitive strategies. Coping mechanisms are thoughts and behaviors that can be used to overcome or manage stressful situations.

(61) (D) Problem-focused coping is characterized by the search for a higher meaning from the situation that might improve one's life in the future.

This is false. Problem-focused coping is characterized by active efforts to cope with information, planning, and positive reframing. The strategies that the individual uses aim to change the situation. An example of problem-focused coping is when someone reads about a problematic topic and creates strategies to overcome the situation based on available information.

(62) (B) Psychopathology and neuroses.

Defense mechanisms are unconscious psychological strategies that an individual uses when faced with a situation that can cause anxiety, depression, or distress. You can think of them as shields against bursts of affect and emotion. Defense mechanisms can be necessary when a person needs to adjust to a reality that cannot be immediately integrated. Excessive use of defense mechanisms is associated with psychopathology and neuroses such as anxiety, phobias, and obsessions.

(63) (A) Denial.

In this case, the patient is unable to cope with the loss and grief due to the death of her son. She refuses the reality of what happened. Denial is a defense mechanism that occurs when an individual denies the facts of objective reality that may be too much to handle. People who are in denial dismiss external reality. For example, denial may be used by an individual who has a serious substance abuse problem but refuses to admit it to themselves and others.

(64) (D) Projection.

This patient is unable to accept his insecurities about his appearance, and he projects those feelings onto other people. This defense mechanism serves to protect the person's self-concept. By projecting unwanted traits onto other people, he denies the existence of these traits in himself.

(65) (D) Regression.

When individuals are faced with a stressful situation, they might revert to an earlier stage of development, like psychological time travel. For example, someone who has lost a pet might start to display behavior normally seen in children. They might start to scream, kick, bite, wet the bed, or throw temper tantrums.

(66) (A) Conversion.

This patient has transferred the anxiety about graduation, moving, and leaving his girlfriend into physical symptoms that cannot be attributed to a medical cause. Conversion is the transformation of intolerable psychiatric symptoms into physical symptoms that cannot be explained by an underlying medical cause or injury. This defense mechanism might cause conversion disorder.

(67) (B) Introjection.

Introjection involves the imitation of someone else's personality traits. Behaviors, thoughts, and characteristics of other people are internalized in the person's self-concept. Freud believed that superegos developed through introjection.

(68) (D) Identification with the aggressor.

This defense mechanism occurs when a victim adopts the behavior of an aggressor in an attempt to avoid abuse and induce empathy. When a victim identifies with the aggressor, they adopt their negative traits.

(69) (A) Jennifer has developed splitting.

Jennifer sees Claire as all good or all bad based on how much her emotional needs are being met. When Claire disappoints her and fails to meet her needs by not going to the theater, Jennifer sees her as all bad. Splitting is commonly seen in borderline personality disorder. It is a failure to recognize the positive and negative characteristics of a person or situation due to conflicting emotions. This results in black-or-white thinking.

(70) (D) Repression.

This defense mechanism is seen in people who have survived a traumatic event but have no recollection of it, even though they did not lose consciousness while it was happening.

(71) (C) Dissociation.

Harry avoids uncomfortable feelings with excessive daydreaming. This defense mechanism is called dissociation. Dissociation occurs when a person copes with stress by detaching from themselves (depersonalization) or the environment around them (derealization). Dissociation also includes a break in memory formation as a protection against high stress. This may cause amnesia or a fragmented sense of self. Excessive daydreaming is an example of dissociation.

(72) (D) Anticipation.

Anticipation is a defense mechanism that consists of efforts to solve the problem before it arises. People who use anticipation predict future problematic events and act accordingly. An example of anticipation would be a student who, to prepare for a difficult exam, practices the hardest questions.

(73) (D) Overcoming perceived weaknesses by emphasizing strengths in other areas.

Compensation as a defense mechanism involves an individual attempting to make up for perceived deficiencies or weaknesses in one area by focusing on and developing strengths in another. This helps to protect the individual's self-esteem and reduce feelings of inadequacy.

(74) (A) Displacement.

Displacement is the transfer of an emotional impulse from one entity to another. Marie displaces the impulse from an unacceptable target—the policeman—to her dog, a more suitable target.

(75) (D) Rationalization.

Adam is using rationalization. In order to avoid disappointment because he could not buy his favorite chocolate, he minimizes the situation and says, "I wanted to try another one either way." Rationalization occurs when someone tries to justify uncomfortable feelings, thoughts, or behaviors through logical explanations.

(76) (A) Reaction formation.

This child is using reaction formation. Reaction formation occurs when someone behaves in the opposite way of what they're truly feeling. This is a conscious way to overcompensate for the unconsciously unacceptable or uncomfortable feelings.

(77) (D) Intellectualization.

Beth is using intellectualization. When faced with a stressful situation, someone who uses intellectualization will start to overanalyze and excessively think about the situation, gather facts, and draw conclusions. Intellectualization puts a distance between a person and their emotions. An example of intellectualization is when someone who discovers they have an illness starts to research everything about the illness instead of showing emotion.

(78) (C) Sublimation.

Derrick is using sublimation. Sublimation is a defense mechanism that is similar to displacement. It occurs when uncomfortable emotions are transformed into constructive behaviors. An example of sublimation is when someone who has uncontrollable anger issues starts a high-intensity sport.

(79) (B) Suppression.

Suppression is similar to repression, but the difference is that while repression is an unconscious process, suppression is a process in which a person consciously chooses to suppress certain uncomfortable or unacceptable thoughts and feelings. An example of suppression is someone who has survived a very traumatic event and keeps having intrusive thoughts about it. They choose to consciously suppress the intrusive thoughts so they can focus on the task at hand.

(80) (D) Basic information about the patient.

The initial interview begins with basic information about the patient (name, age, marital status, sex, race or ethnicity, and occupation). The second part of the interview is the identification of the source and reliability of the information. The third part is the chief complaint, which consists of the main symptom bothering the patient, written in the patient's own words. An example is "I feel very anxious."

(81) (C) History of present illness.

The history of the present illness is a chronological description of the course of current symptoms. This section begins with an open-ended question, such as "What brought you here today?" Information that should be obtained includes the type of symptoms, how long they have been present, the severity, fluctuations in the severity or nature, the presence or absence of stressors, and factors that alleviate or worsen symptoms.

(82) (C) Take a detailed past psychiatric history.

The psychiatric mental health nurse practitioner should gather detailed information about previous psychiatric illnesses, their evolution over the patient's life, prior episodes of the current illness, and the frequency and severity of previous episodes. Detailed information about past treatment should also be included, such as inpatient treatment (voluntary or involuntary hospitalization), outpatient treatment (psychotherapy, day treatment, partial hospitalization), medications, electroconvulsive therapy, and other treatment modalities.

(83) (A) Use a nonjudgmental manner to obtain accurate information.

Questions about substance use, abuse, and addictions should be asked in a nonjudgmental manner in order for the psychiatric mental health nurse practitioner to obtain accurate information. The history should include what type of substances have been used, the route of use, frequency and amount, tolerance, withdrawal symptoms, need for increasing the amounts, the impact on social interactions, and legal consequences.

(84) (B) A medical condition cannot be precipitated by the treatment of a psychiatric illness.

This is false. A medical condition can be precipitated by the treatment of a psychiatric illness, such as metabolic syndrome caused by second-generation antipsychotics. A medical condition can worsen the symptoms of a psychiatric illness, like when a patient with anxiety is diagnosed with cancer. A medical condition can also mimic a psychiatric illness (hypothyroidism mimics major depressive disorder). Because of this, the past medical history should include the presence of any medical conditions, surgical history, and treatment.

(85) (D) Relationships and marriage history.

Relationships and marriage history reflect the patient's ability to develop and maintain interpersonal relationships. The childhood history consists of information about the patient's home environment and friendships. School history contains information on the patient's academic success or difficulties, learning disorders, extracurricular activities, and behavioral history. Work history contains information about the types of jobs the patient has worked, how frequently the patient changes jobs, work performance, and relationships with authorities and coworkers.

(86) (C) Mental status examination.

The mental status examination is an objective tool that gathers information about areas of mental functioning and signs and symptoms of psychiatric disease. The examination begins from the moment the patient enters the room during the first interaction. The information is gathered from observation. It reveals information about the current mental state of the patient and can be used to monitor progress over time.

(87) (D) Appearance and behavior.

In the section about appearance and behavior, health practitioners provide a description of the patient's general description—how they look and behave. Does the patient look like their age? What are they wearing, and is it appropriate? Do they look like they take care of their hygiene and grooming? Are there any distinguishing features such as tattoos, scars, or disfigurations? Is the patient cooperative, uncooperative, agitated, disinhibited, disinterested, etc.?

(88) (A) Pressured speech.

Speed of speech is an important element since it can provide diagnostic clues. Slow speech is associated with depression. Rapid and pressured speech can be seen in mania or hypomania. The amount of speech can be increased (mania, hypomania, ADHD) or decreased (depression, psychosis, thought blocking). Tone and volume of speech can be described as dysphoric, irritable, loud, anxious, quiet, timid, childlike, or angry.

(89) (A) Incongruent, depressed.

This patient reports that her mood (internal emotional experience) is depressed, but she laughs hysterically, which means her affect is incongruent with her mood. Affect is the external expression of the patient's mood or what it appears to be to the person who examines the patient. Congruency refers to the compatibility of the affect with the patient's mood or thought content.

(90) (A) Goal-directed.

The thought process refers to the formulation, organization, and expression of thoughts. It does not take into account the content. The normal thought process is goal-directed, linear, and organized. Examples of abnormal thought processes include flight of ideas, circumstantiality, clang association, thought blocking, tangential thoughts, loose thoughts or associations, perseveration, and derailment.

(91) (D) Delusion.

Delusions are false, fixed beliefs that can be bizarre (out of the realm of possibility) and nonbizzarre (not out of the realm of possibility but still not true). Delusions can be categorized as grandiose, jealous, persecutory, somatic, and erotomanic. Perceptual disturbances are illusions, hallucinations, depersonalization, and derealization.

(92) (C) Cognition.

Cognition consists of alertness, orientation, concentration, memory, calculation, knowledge, abstract reasoning, insight, and judgment. To test alertness, observe the patient's ability to function. Ask patients general questions like their name, location, etc. This tests orientation. To test concentration, have patients count backward by seven from 100.

(93) (B) Insight.

Insight refers to the patient's comprehension of the existence of his psychiatric illness. Insight can be absent, partial, or full. A patient who is psychotic may say, "I am aware that there are no aliens out to get me, but I can hear their voices even though I know they're not there." This patient has insight even though he has a severe psychiatric disease.

(94) (A) Previous suicide attempts.

The strongest risk factors for suicidality are previous suicide attempts and the presence of a psychiatric disorder. The psychiatric mental health nurse practitioner can use screening instruments to identify patients who are at risk. Screening instruments are combined with clinical assessment of risk. The suicide assessment is done in all patients.

(95) (C) Perseveration.

Perseveration refers to the failure of the patient to move on to other topics despite the clinician's attempt to change the fixated topic of conversation. Examples of abnormal thought processes include flight of ideas, circumstantiality, clang association, thought blocking, tangential thoughts, loose thoughts or associations, perseveration, and derailment. For example, a patient with a flight of ideas rapidly moves from one topic to another. The ideas are logically connected, but they are hard to keep up with. In loose associations, there is rapid movement from one thought to another, but the thoughts are not connected logically.

(96) (A) Ask patients openly if they have suicidal thoughts.

The suicide assessment is done in all patients. It includes prior history, family history of suicide attempts, and history of completed suicides. The patient should be asked about current ideation, plan, and intent. Prior attempts should be assessed for potential triggers and their lethality risk. It is necessary to ask patients about current thoughts of suicide and intent. Patients should be asked what has previously prevented them from ending their life.

(97) (D) Treats this information as important since it is relevant to the patient's suicide risk.

It is necessary to keep preventative factors in mind since their loss might increase the risk of suicide. For example, a patient who says their pet is keeping them alive may be at an increased suicide risk if the pet gets lost or dies. Factors that increase the risk of suicide include male sex, advanced age, single marital status (or widower), lower socioeconomic status, unemployment, depression, schizophrenia, alcohol or drug abuse/dependence, and distressing life events.

(98) (C) Family history of psychiatric disorders.

A family history of psychiatric disorders is not part of the risk assessment. Areas that are assessed include the risk of suicide, self-harm, danger to others, vulnerability to exploitation, the likelihood of substance abuse, noncompliance with treatment, homelessness, and risk of self-neglect.

(99) (D) Hepatitis C test.

In young patients who have a history of drug abuse, Hepatitis B, C, and HIV tests should be ordered. Tests that are done when the patient presents for the first time include hepatic, renal, and thyroid function, complete blood count, and calcium and phosphate levels. If a patient is suspected to have organic cerebral pathology, other diagnostic tests, such as CT, MRI, EEG, etc., should be ordered.

(100) (D) Client-centered care.

Client-centered care, also called patient-centered care, is a healthcare model that is focused on making the patient feel involved in their treatment and care journey. With client-centered care, patients receive highly personalized care. The goal of client-centered care is to empower and educate patients, encourage patients to make decisions about their treatment plans, create individualized plans, and improve patient outcomes.

(101) (B) Use a holistic approach and consider the well-being of the patient as a whole instead of isolating the illness.

Nurses who are educated in client-centered care use a holistic approach and consider the well-being of the patient as a whole instead of isolating the illness. The core concept of client-centered care is a focus on the individual who is experiencing the physical or mental health issue and all aspects of their functioning, rather than just treating the disease.

(102) (D) Should be welcoming and safe.

The first appointment at the psychiatrist can intimidate patients. The psychiatric mental health nurse practitioner should make sure the initial interaction between the patient and a healthcare provider is in a safe, comfortable environment. This is particularly emphasized in patients who are in a state of agitation, panic, psychosis, etc.

(103) (A) Respect for the patient's preferences, needs, and values.

The psychiatric mental health nurse practitioner should get to know patients on an individual level and recognize their strengths, beliefs, perspectives, needs, and values. Patients should be treated as an active participant in their treatment plan. Information about the patient's priorities should be obtained. The patient, the family, and caregivers should be informed of the treatment plan, prognosis, and outcomes.

(104) (A) Transitions between different providers in different phases of treatment should be smooth and not cause confusion and stress.

The medical team should be organized and coordinated. Coordinated treatment enables a smooth and productive recovery. This is especially important for patients who need various types of care. Disruptive, disorganized care may cause poor outcomes. The psychiatric mental health nurse practitioner should assess the patient's need for different services, both formal and informal. Care management and referrals should be provided as needed.

(105) (D) Show empathy and reassure the patient.

The psychiatric mental health nurse practitioner should consider the patient's emotional well-being and provide care in an empathetic environment. Patients should be offered sensitivity and reassurance. Psychiatric disorders have an impact on the emotional well-being of patients. Often, when a patient is diagnosed with a psychiatric disorder, they are faced with stigma. The disorder might cause them to lose their job or a significant other.

(106) (D) The patient should not have any responsibilities in the treatment journey.

This is false. Responsibility is one of the elements of client-centered care. The patient should be a proactive participant in the healthcare journey. The psychiatric mental health nurse practitioner should enable patients to take care of themselves by teaching them the necessary skills. Patients should perform as many tasks as they are able. This will increase patients' self-esteem and develop their skills. The psychiatric mental health nurse practitioner should recognize patient boundaries and not push them too far.

(107) (A) Psychopharmacology treatment plan.

A psychopharmacology treatment plan is part of the therapeutic interventions for medical management of the patient's illness, and therefore, it is not a part of the principles of client-centered care.

(108) (A) Inform the patient of the increased prolactin levels.

Patients should be enabled to be proactive in their treatment journey. The psychiatric mental health practitioner should educate patients on the steps in the care plan, their lab results, physical findings, expected effects of medications, adverse effects, etc.

(109) (B) The nurse encourages the client to participate in decisions about their care and respects their preferences and values.

This approach ensures that care is tailored to each client, and fosters a therapeutic partnership between the nurse and the client. It promotes autonomy, improves client satisfaction, and can lead to better health outcomes by aligning care with what is most meaningful and beneficial to the client.

(110) (A) Inform the patient that the information shared during the interview is confidential.

To make sure the patient feels safe disclosing information, the nurse should inform him of the confidentiality of the provider-patient relationship.

(111) (C) Be empathetic toward John and provide comfort and reassurance. Explain that the benefits of treatment outweigh the cons.

Psychiatric disorders have an impact on the emotional well-being of patients. The psychiatric mental health nurse practitioner should be able to address patients' fears, such as the impact of their disease on their life, the financial costs of the disease, and anxieties related to the side effects of medications.

(112) (C) Most individuals feel as if they are completely involved in their mental health treatment.

This is false. Some reports suggest that 60% of individuals feel as if they are not completely involved in their treatment. Some studies suggest that psychiatrists inaccurately overestimate their collaboration. Currently, psychiatry uses a bio-psycho-social model that is considered client-centered.

(113) (B) Human rights and relevant legislation.

Healthcare providers in psychiatry are often required to restrict the individual freedoms of patients to achieve the best clinical outcome. Clinicians must achieve a balance between respect for the patient's human rights and the provision of the best care. Healthcare providers must be knowledgeable about human rights and relevant legislation. They should always respect people's human rights and wishes and treat patients with dignity.

(114) (D) Might have to choose a treatment that is not the best according to current evidence-based medicine.

The patient's history, values, circumstances, and strengths influence the clinician's decision-making process about diagnosis, support, and management plan. In client-centered care, the clinician develops the management plan in collaboration with the patient.

(115) (D) Aims to improve work satisfaction and reduce burnout levels.

The client-centered care approach aims to improve the lives of healthcare providers. Psychiatric healthcare providers are at risk of burnout. This influences both the clinicians' well-being and quality of life, as well as the clinical outcomes.

(116) (C) Client-centered care emphasizes guidelines and protocols.

This is false. The practice of evidence-based medicine incorporates clinical guidelines and protocols. In a client-centered care approach, the clinical decision process should not be based on blind use of guidelines and protocols. Collaboration between healthcare providers and patients should ensure that care is tailored to the individual's specific situation and needs.

(117) (A) The patient's literacy level and preferred learning style.

When you are providing patient education, you should consider the patient's literacy level and preferred learning style. Tailoring education to the patient's capabilities and preferences ensures that the information is comprehensible and retainable.

(118) (D) Intelligence.

Primary individual factors include the age of the individual, intelligence, previous learning, anxiety, and motivation. Intelligence has many theories and definitions. It is the capacity of the individual to learn and use new information. A combination of inherent and acquired capabilities influences the individual's intelligence level.

(119) (C) New knowledge is built upon previous knowledge, and new and old knowledge are connected.

Learning has a hierarchical component, which means that new knowledge is built upon previous knowledge, and new and old knowledge are connected. The hierarchical nature has an especially big influence on children since learning is largely dependent on age and maturation. For the individual to learn, they must be ready to do so.

(120) (B) A bachelor's degree in organic chemistry.

A patient with a bachelor's degree in organic chemistry has a high level of education in a complex topic. This will enable them to grasp complex topics more easily. The amount of knowledge a person has learned throughout their life will significantly contribute to the ease and speed of learning new material. This is especially true if the new material is related to something that was previously learned.

(121) (D) Anxiety creates hopelessness, which can make the person unwilling to learn new material.

How much anxiety an individual experiences is another factor that impacts the process of learning. Individuals may feel afraid of failure. They may lack self-confidence and have a low degree of self-efficacy. All these factors impact the person's ability to learn. Anxiety can elicit various responses. For example, someone who fears failure may start to feel hopeless, which can result in the person being reluctant to learn new content.

(122) (D) Passivity and resistance.

How you present the material is an important factor in the learning process. Even though there are variations in people's abilities and motivations to learn, there are certain methods that can maximize the effectiveness and efficiency of learning for the majority of people. These methods have an impact on recall, transfer, and retention. The most important methods include active participation, distribution of practice, whole versus part, and knowledge of results.

(123) (A) Asks questions and makes comments.

Active participation increases individuals' ability to learn from both cognitive and psychomotor tasks. When they take an active role in the learning process, people can better understand, develop their skills, and increase retention. When people actively participate, they pay attention, search for patterns and relationships in the material, make comments, ask questions, think about the content, and practice skills.

(124) (D) People learn better when they pay attention only to the discrete parts, not the entirety of the material.

This is false. People learn better when they have an image of the whole before learning something in its entirety. When they review the entire task first, they are able to understand where each part fits and what its use is. To help learners, you should break down a task into smaller manageable units. This will make it easier for learners to focus and avoid overwhelm.

(125) (B) There is no need to inform people about their test results since that might discourage them.

This is false. When you inform people about their results and give them constructive feedback, this facilitates the learning process. People feel encouraged to get better when they receive input on how they are doing. Input enables people to acknowledge their strengths and identify and correct potential errors.

(126) (A) It increases the motivation of the learner.

Motivation for learning is increased when the material has meaning. Individuals can make associations with material they have previously learned, with their needs or drives, or with emotional content. To help people see associations, organize the material into conceptual categories.

(127) (C) Vertical transfer.

Transfer is divided into horizontal and vertical. Vertical transfer occurs when the individual uses old concepts to understand or learn concepts with increased complexity. Horizontal transfer occurs when a new task is performed at the same level of complexity as an old task. The theory of identical elements states that transfer occurs from one learning to another when the two materials have common elements.

(128) (B) The second (contemplative) stage of change.

In the second stage, patients start to consider change, but they are still not ready to take action. In the first stage (pre-contemplative), patients are not aware that they have a problem and may not be ready to act. In the third (action) stage, patients start to practice behavioral change and learn how to maintain it. In the fourth (maintenance) stage, patients reinforce the learned behavior, and it becomes a part of their everyday life.

(129) (D) Teach the patient about how addiction affects her life.

In this situation, the patient is not aware that she has a problem, and therefore, psychoeducation should increase that awareness. The interventions that the clinician makes will be most effective if they match the patient's readiness to learn.

(130) (A) Ask if they prefer to learn during the day or at night.

Assessing patients' learning styles will help you match your teaching strategies to their learning styles, which will make learning more effective. You can ask patients which time of the day they prefer to learn, if they enjoy reading or prefer video formats, and if they want the material to be explained to them before they read it or after. You can ask patients if they have any problems that would prevent them from learning new material in the current moment.

(131) (B) Learning objectives are long term.

This is false. Learning objectives are short term, attainable, and measurable. Achieving goals can be made easier if they are broken down into learning objectives. An example of a learning objective is "After this meeting, the patient will be able to identify the symptoms of depression." This is a step toward a larger goal. When learning objectives are developed, measurable terms, such as explain, list, or demonstrate, should be used.

(132) (B) List of prescribed medications.

To assess the patient's learning style, ask them directly or gather information from the family, other healthcare staff, and checklists and questionnaires. Conversations with family members can help you understand the patient's home situation and assess whether the family is supportive of the patient's wish to change their behavior. Collaboration with the healthcare team can provide valuable information about what type of teaching strategies to use.

(133) (A) Assess the patient's learning needs.

Assessment of the patient's learning needs is the first process in patient education.

(134) (A) Readiness to learn.

The clinician should develop goals for the individual or psychoeducational group. The goals should be direct, clear, and specific. They should consider the needs, readiness, and motivations of the learners. Sometimes this can be hard to achieve if the clinician does not have a lot of information about the individuals or the participants before the first meeting.

(135) (C) New material interferes with the retrieval of old material.

Retroactive inhibition happens when new material interferes with the retrieval of old material. The trace decay theory of forgetting states that people retain and strengthen memories they use, while the memories that are not used gradually fade away. The interference theory states that proactive inhibition is a cause of forgetting that occurs when previous learning interferes with the learning of new material.

(136) (C) The educator's intelligence level.

The educator's intelligence level does not influence the retention of learning. Retention is increased when the material is thoroughly learned, the material has meaning for the learner, the learner uses the material after learning it, and there are no intervening situations that are traumatic enough to interfere.

(137) (C) Culture.

Culture can be defined as a way of life in a specific society that consists of shared patterns of belief, knowledge, and feelings that influence people's behavior. These patterns are passed down from generation to generation. Ethnicity refers to a common identity in people because of a shared heritage. Culture and ethnicity affect human behavior.

(138) (A) Stereotyping.

Nurses must obtain knowledge on cultural concepts and ethnicity to work with people with different cultural backgrounds. However, they should be careful not to assume that all people from the same cultural or ethnic groups exhibit the same behavior. This is called stereotyping. There are many variations and subcultures that exist within a culture. These variations may be due to status, residence, religion, education, ethnic background, etc. Every patient's uniqueness must be appreciated.

(139) (D) Culturally competent care.

Culturally competent care is a way to minimize misunderstandings that may arise between healthcare providers and patients because of cultural diversity. In the US, a large number of residents are immigrants, descendants of immigrants, or foreign-born residents.

(140) (D) Healthcare providers are allowed to use slang if the patient chooses to use it.

This is false. Healthcare educators should be educated on important issues as well as the proper usage of terms. But sometimes patients may use slang terms such as homo, queer, dyke, or fag when describing themselves or their partners. It is important to know that these terms are considered derogatory when used by a healthcare provider.

(141) (C) A person who is in between genders and has both male and female characteristics.

Androgyny or gender neutrality means a person is in between genders and has both male and female characteristics. A person who is attracted to both females and males is bisexual. The individual's sense of gender, which may be different from the assigned sex at birth, is gender identity. A person who is attracted to members of the opposite sex is heterosexual.

(142) (C) Gender expression.

Gender expression is the appearance, social behavior, style, or mannerisms associated with masculinity or femininity.

(143) (D) Previous positive experiences with clinicians.

LGBTQ patients may have had previous traumatic experiences with other clinicians, which may be a challenge for new providers who work with them. Other challenges include difficulties discussing sexual health-related problems, lack of familiarity with gender modification surgery, forgetting to use gender-neutral terms (e.g., significant other, partner), patients' reluctance to share sexual practices, use of language that is derogatory, and making assumptions about a patient based on their appearance.

(144) (C) Lesbian women, gay men, and bisexual people have a lower chance of dying by suicide.

This is false. LGBTQ patients have a higher risk of mental health issues compared to their heterosexual peers. They also have a higher chance of suffering from depression and have higher rates of substance abuse, which may be due to the stress caused by homophobia and discrimination. Adolescents who are a part of a sexual and gender minority have a higher chance of suicide.

(145) (C) CAGE.

The CAGE questionnaire is a widely used screening tool for alcohol use disorders. It consists of four questions that help identify potential problems with alcohol. A score of two or more "yes" answers suggests significant alcohol problems and indicates the need for further evaluation.

(146) (B) Reserved and silent.

There are 574 American Indian tribes and Alaska Native groups currently recognized by the federal government. Native Americans may sometimes appear as reserved and silent people who do not express much emotion. Some Native American cultures believe that private thoughts should be kept to oneself. Some Native Americans consider the classical handshake to be too aggressive. Eye contact is sometimes considered to be rude in some Native American cultures.

(147) (D) Shaman.

Religion and health are combined in Native American culture. The healer is sometimes called the shaman. The shaman uses many practices, such as the use of crystals to diagnose disease, songs, healing ceremonies, and plants, roots, and herbs with healing properties.

(148) (A) Addiction to alcohol.

Alcoholism is a significant issue in Native American culture. Native Americans have a higher risk of illness and premature death from diabetes, tuberculosis, heart disease, suicide, pneumonia, influence, homicide, and alcoholism. They have higher rates of depression, spouse and child abuse, and automobile accidents.

(149) (C) Generativity vs. Stagnation.

According to Erik Erikson's stages of psychosocial development, a 45-year-old individual is usually in the stage of Generativity vs. Stagnation. This stage, which occurs during middle adulthood (approximately ages 40 to 65), involves individuals striving to contribute to society and help guide the next generation through activities such as parenting, mentoring, and community involvement. Success in this stage leads to feelings of usefulness and accomplishment, while failure results in shallow involvement in the world and a sense of stagnation.

(150) (D) Some Asian Americans consider eye contact disrespectful.

People from Asian American cultures may consider raising one's voice a sign of losing control, and physical contact during conversation could be seen as unacceptable. Eye contact may be seen as a lack of respect.

Test 2: Questions

(1) Which of the following is not an element of a treatment plan?

(A) Identifying and background information.

(B) Goals and Objectives.

(C) Trauma history.

(D) List of problems.

(2) The first part of a treatment plan is called:

(A) Presenting problem.

(B) Identifying and basic information.

(C) Referral source and reason for referral.

(D) Problem list.

(3) The person who referred the patient for treatment is identified in which section of a treatment plan?

(A) Problem list.

(B) Presenting problem.

(C) Identifying and background information.

(D) Referral source and reason for referral.

(4) Which of the following descriptions presents the patient's main complaint most appropriately?

(A) "The patient suffers from depression."

(B) "The patient suffers from antisocial personality disorder."

(C) "The patient has been feeling on edge lately. He worries that his wife might leave him because he lost his job. He cannot fall asleep at night. He feels hopeless and lost."

(D) "The patient has many somatoform complaints."

(5) Which of the following statements regarding the problem list of the treatment plan is false?

(A) The problems should be presented in a way that shows how they manifest in the patient and their life.

(B) The problems should significantly impact the patient's daily life and ability to function (e.g., work, school, social, and family).

(C) The problems should be solvable with a health intervention.

(D) The problems should be described generally, e.g., "school problems."

(6) When assessing a patient's developmental history, which of the following aspects is most critical for understanding potential mental health issues?

(A) Academic performance.

(B) Physical growth milestones.

(C) Family dynamics.

(D) Sleep patterns.

(7) Which of the following questions should be asked first when prioritizing the problem list?

(A) What problem most impacts the patient's life?

(B) Is there a problem that poses a danger to the patient or others?

(C) Is there a problem that blocks solutions to other problems?

(D) Is there a problem that is easily solvable?

(8) Which of the following describes a lower-priority problem which can be addressed later in treatment?

(A) A problem that, if treated, might destabilize the patient.

(B) A problem that will jeopardize the therapy.

(C) A problem that will block solutions to other issues.

(D) The problem the patient is most committed to solving.

(9) A patient-related factor that limits the length of treatment is:

(A) Limitations of a healthcare plan.

(B) Reduced practice hours.

(C) Permanent closing of the practice.

(D) Temporary closing of the practice.

(10) Diagnoses based on accepted diagnostic classification systems make communication easier between healthcare providers (and other parties). The most commonly used diagnostic classification system is:

(A) DSM-IV.

(B) ICD-10.

(C) ICD-11.

(D) DSM-V.

(11) Which of the following characteristics is not usually associated with well-formed goals and objectives in a treatment plan?

(A) Specific.

(B) Measurable.

(C) Abstract.

(D) Time-limited.

(12) The S in the SMART goals approach stands for:

(A) Short-term.

(B) Subsequent.

(C) Safe.

(D) Specific.

(13) Which of the following criteria of the SMART goals approach gauges progress?

(A) Specific.

(B) Measurable.

(C) Achievable.

(D) Realistic.

(14) A twenty-three-year-old female patient with chronic schizophrenia is treated with olanzapine and has gained twenty pounds in the past two months. She wants to exercise three hours daily to lose twenty pounds in the next week. Which of the following is true for her goal?

(A) It is achievable.

(B) It is reasonable.

(C) It is realistic.

(D) It is unachievable in the specified timeline.

(15) A clinician must determine whether a goal is achievable. This means a patient can accomplish the goal with the given circumstances and resources. If the goal is achievable, they should establish whether the patient can accomplish it within a reasonable timeline. The next step is to determine if the goal is:

(A) Realistic.

(B) Specific.

(C) Measurable.

(D) Time-bound.

(16) What does the T stand for in the SMART goals approach?

(A) Treatment plan.

(B) Teaching.

(C) Time-bound.

(D) Treating clinician.

(17) The treatment plan will be used mainly by:

(A) The patient.

(B) The treating clinician.

(C) Insurers.

(D) Third-party stakeholders.

(18) The treatment plan can serve as a source of reassurance for:

(A) Third-party stakeholders.

(B) Insurers.

(C) The patient.

(D) The treating clinician.

(19) Which of the following parties must be provided with evidence that the treatment is medically necessary?

(A) Third-party stakeholders.

(B) Insurers.

(C) The patient.

(D) The treating clinician.

(20) Other parties may have a stake in the patient's treatment, depending on their current life circumstances. Third-party stakeholders would be most interested in:

(A) The patient's motivation for completing treatment.

(B) Whether the treatment is short-term or long-term.

(C) Whether the patient is a danger to others.

(D) The patient's will to engage in treatment.

(21) Which of the following is not a part of the cognitive triad which is the basis for cognitive behavioral therapy?

(A) The beliefs people have about themselves.

(B) The beliefs people have about the world around them.

(C) The beliefs people have about spirituality.

(D) The beliefs people have about the future.

(22) According to the cognitive model, emotional distress and negative experiences can cause the development of negative cognitive patterns. Their development is associated with many psychiatric disorders, such as:

(A) Depression.

(B) Dissociative identity disorder.

(C) Schizophrenia.

(D) Bipolar disorder.

(23) A thirty-five-year-old female patient refuses to go to social events. She says, “I am uglier than all the other women, and it is pointless to show up since nobody wants to talk to me either way.” How can the psychiatric mental health nurse practitioner help her?

(A) Prescribe an antipsychotic for her delusions.

(B) Order an MRI to check for a brain tumor that may be the cause of her feelings.

(C) Order a thyroid function test to check for low thyroid hormone levels.

(D) Help her elicit automatic thoughts and test their validity with cognitive behavioral therapy techniques.

(24) A fifty-five-year-old male patient struggles with anxiety caused by excessive perfectionism in work performance. He worries that he might get fired if he fails at a task. He says, “If they notice anything wrong, they will know I'm inadequate, and I'll lose my job.” This patient has:

(A) A hopeful view of the future.

(B) A negative belief about himself.

(C) A negative belief about his family.

(D) An appropriate reaction to the circumstances.

(25) Which of the following is not a cognitive technique of cognitive behavioral therapy?

(A) Elicite automatic thoughts.

(B) Test the validity of maladaptive assumptions.

(C) Identify maladaptive assumptions.

(D) Journal daily activities.

(26) A twenty-five-year-old female patient with depression complains of having no friends. She believes that nobody will love her if she is not perfect. She tries to compensate for her low self-esteem by people-pleasing. She hopes people will stay if she fulfills all of their needs. How can the psychiatric mental health nurse practitioner help this patient?

(A) Prescribe a benzodiazepine to calm her anxiety.

(B) Teach her to identify and test maladaptive assumptions.

(C) Show her social media sites where she can find friends.

(D) Refer her to a neurologist.

(27) Which of the following statements regarding the recovery model is false?

(A) It is based on the assumption that people can heal from mental illness.

(B) Hope is the driving force behind recovery.

(C) Patients with psychiatric diseases do not need additional empowerment.

(D) Spirituality can bring hope and meaning to a person's life after they have survived a stressful event.

(28) Which of the following is not an indication for cognitive behavioral therapy?

(A) A patient with depression who believes he is bad at everything he does.

(B) A patient with panic disorder who believes that he can easily get hurt and break his leg.

(C) A patient with schizophrenia who believes that ghosts are after him.

(D) A patient with OCD who has trouble believing in the fidelity of partners.

(29) Which of the following is most effective for improving interpersonal relationships of patients with borderline personality disorder?

(A) Cognitive Behavioral Therapy.

(B) Dialectical Behavior Therapy.

(C) Psychodynamic Therapy.

(D) Electroconvulsive Therapy.

(30) Which of the following types of psychotherapy can be used to treat all mental disorders?

(A) Psychoanalytic psychotherapy.

(B) Psychodynamic psychotherapy.

(C) Supportive psychotherapy.

(D) Interpersonal psychotherapy.

(31) The main goal of supportive psychotherapy is to:

(A) Help patients through difficult times and situations.

(B) Create a supportive environment where patients can learn new social skills.

(C) Teach patients to identify maladaptive assumptions that cause them to engage in maladaptive behaviors.

(D) Provide insight into interpersonal conflicts.

(32) During supportive psychotherapy, therapists teach patients:

(A) How to deal with conflicts in their close relationships.

(B) Specific coping techniques.

(C) Cognitive and behavioral techniques to identify and test automatic thoughts.

(D) Breathing techniques and mindfulness to reduce anxiety.

(33) Which of the following is not an advantage of group therapy?

(A) It provides a supportive environment that enables patients to improve their interactions with others.

(B) It teaches patients to cope with difficult experiences, adjustment periods, and situations.

(C) It helps patients change maladaptive cognitions by testing the inaccuracy of their maladaptive cognitive structures.

(D) It requires therapists to undergo extensive psychotherapy.

(34) The mental healthcare approach that takes into account the impact of psychological trauma on patients and staff and aims to provide care in a way that will not cause re-traumatization is called:

(A) Client-centered care.

(B) Patient-centered care.

(C) Trauma-informed care.

(D) Staff-centered care.

(35) The psychiatric mental health nurse practitioner can make patients feel comfortable by using:

(A) An assertive body position.

(B) Medical terminology when talking to the patient.

(C) An open and non-threatening body position.

(D) A dominating and strict posture.

(36) A patient on 225 mg Venlafaxine (Effexor) needs to have their blood pressure measured a few times a day. According to the principles of trauma-informed care, the psychiatric mental health nurse practitioner should:

(A) Measure the patient's blood pressure at any time since it is for their own good.

(B) Ask the patient for permission every time before measuring their blood pressure.

(C) Ask the patient for permission only the first time in the morning and explain that their blood pressure will be measured multiple times a day.

(D) There is no need to ask permission to measure the patient's blood pressure since the consequences of not doing so would be catastrophic.

(37) A patient with schizophrenia is hospitalized in the inpatient psychiatric unit. During the morning visit, the nurse and doctor are accompanied by six medical students. The patient looks anxious. The psychiatric mental health nurse practitioner should:

(A) Inform the doctor of the patient's state.

(B) Teach the students about anxiety in psychotic patients.

(C) Increase the dose of olanzapine.

(D) Ask the medical students to leave the room.

(38) A psychiatric mental health nurse practitioner visits a patient with anorexia nervosa for the second time that day. According to the principles of trauma-informed care, how should the nurse announce her visit?

(A) "Hi! It is nice to see you again."

(B) "Hello. How have you been since this morning? Do you feel better?"

(C) "Hi. I know we have met before, but I would like to remind you that I am your mental health nurse and will take care of you during your stay."

(D) "Hi! I am just checking to see if you need anything. How have you been feeling?"

(39) Which of the following statements regarding the principles of trauma-informed care is false?

(A) The psychiatric mental health nurse practitioner should ask for permission before touching patients, even after performing a task multiple times in a day.

(B) When communicating with patients, use clear and straightforward language and avoid medical jargon.

(C) Patients should not be informed of what to expect since that might cause too much anxiety.

(D) The patient should not be responsible for asking others to leave since they may not feel empowered to do so.

(40) Which of the following is a component of the recovery model?

(A) Self-identity.

(B) Behavioral interventions.

(C) ACE score.

(D) Medication management.

(41) Which of the following is not a reason to choose complementary and alternative interventions?

(A) A desire for more control in the decision process.

(B) Low insurance coverage for conventional treatment.

(C) A preference for natural health alternatives.

(D) Lack of side effects of the current medication.

(42) Non-conventional treatments that are added to conventional medical treatment are called:

(A) Alternative interventions.

(B) Complementary interventions.

(C) Integrative methods.

(D) Psychotherapeutic methods.

(43) A nineteen-year-old female patient complains of anhedonia, loss of appetite, and insomnia. She is diagnosed with depression. She says that she does not want to take an antidepressant because she does not believe in them, but she read online that omega-3 can be an effective treatment for depression. Since she prefers to use natural products, she asks the psychiatric mental health nurse practitioner if she thinks this would be a useful treatment for her. How should the nurse practitioner respond?

(A) Agree and confirm that the patient can use omega-3 to treat her depression.

(B) Explain that omega-3 is not an effective monotherapy for depression but can be used in combination with an antidepressant.

(C) Deny her request and insist that she take an antidepressant only.

(D) Prescribe a combination of omega-3 and gingko biloba.

(44) A forty-five-year-old patient with bipolar disorder and primary genetic trimethylaminuria (a genetic disease characterized by fishy body odor) considers adding the supplement Choline to their treatment regimen. They read online that it can be helpful for people with bipolar disorder. How should the psychiatric mental health nurse practitioner respond?

(A) Agree and add Choline to the patient's treatment regimen.

(B) Deny their request and suggest an increase in the dose of the mood stabilizer.

(C) Explain to the patient that he should not take Choline due to his genetic condition.

(D) Explain to the patient that supplements are not helpful for bipolar disorder.

(45) A thirty-four-year-old male patient with major depressive disorder complained of diarrhea and increased temperature. The psychiatric mental health nurse practitioner reviewed his medication and saw that he had been prescribed 60 mg of fluoxetine. She asked whether he had been taking anything else, and the patient reported that he had been taking a supplement called 5-HTP. The psychiatric mental health nurse practitioner:

(A) Immediately discontinues both fluoxetine and 5-HTP.

(B) Increases the dose of fluoxetine.

(C) Increases the dose of 5-HTP.

(D) Discontinues fluoxetine only.

(46) A sixty-seven-year-old female patient is scheduled for a cholecystectomy. Which of the following vitamins should the patient discontinue before her surgery?

(A) Vitamin E.

(B) Vitamin C.

(C) Vitamin D.

(D) Vitamin B6.

(47) A twenty-five-year-old female patient complains of increased irritability, bloating, and depressive mood right before the start of her menstrual cycle. Which of the following supplements are recommended for this patient?

(A) Melatonin.

(B) Vitamin C.

(C) Choline.

(D) Vitamin E.

(48) Which of the following supplements can inhibit ovulation in higher doses?

(A) DHA.

(B) Choline.

(C) Melatonin.

(D) Vitamin D.

(49) A thirty-seven-year-old male patient with bipolar disorder presents in a manic episode. Which of the following combinations could have induced his mania?

(A) Valerian and paroxetine.

(B) Sertraline and St. John's wort.

(C) Gingko and fluoxetine.

(D) Ginseng and olanzapine.

(50) Which of the following herbal products should not be used with alcohol or CNS depressants due to their sedative effects?

(A) Ginseng.

(B) Gingko biloba.

(C) Valerian.

(D) St. John's wort.

(51) A twenty-two-year-old male patient diagnosed with depression complains of sexual dysfunction since he started treatment with sertraline. He also complains of poor memory and concentration. Which of the following herbal products can potentially alleviate his symptoms?

(A) Ginseng.

(B) Valerian.

(C) St. John's wort.

(D) Gingko.

(52) A fifty-six-year-old patient is scheduled for an elective surgical procedure. Which of the following products could increase his risk of bleeding?

(A) Ginseng.

(B) Vitamin C.

(C) Valerian.

(D) Chamomile.

(53) A seventy-year-old male patient who has Parkinson's disease is treated with levodopa. Which of the following supplements is contraindicated for use in this patient?

(A) Lavender.

(B) Ginseng.

(C) Valerian.

(D) Kava kava.

(54) Which of the following supplements is used in aromatherapy to treat anxiety?

(A) Kava kava.

(B) Lavender.

(C) Ginseng.

(D) Valerian.

(55) The psychiatric mental health nurse practitioner should inform patients of the pros and cons of using natural products as a part of their care. Which of the following patients is less likely to benefit from adding a natural product?

(A) A fifty-six-year-old male patient who prefers natural products because of his religious practices.

(B) A twenty-three-year-old female patient who has tried multiple SSRIs to treat depression but cannot tolerate the side effects.

(C) A forty-five-year-old patient with schizophrenia who has his illness under control with 4 mg risperidone.

(D) A seventeen-year-old patient with an inadequate nutrient intake and vitamin deficiency.

(56) Which of the following medications is most likely to cause somnolence as a side effect in patients who are being treated for anxiety?

(A) Fluoxetine.

(B) Lorazepam.

(C) Buspirone.

(D) Sertraline.

(57) The deliberate organization of patient care activities between healthcare professionals is called:

(A) Educational conceptualization.

(B) Care coordination.

(C) Communication.

(D) Ethical consideration.

(58) The main goal of care coordination in mental health is to make sure that patients:

(A) Receive the right services at the right time.

(B) Feel safe in their environment.

(C) Have an effective patient-provider relationship.

(D) Increase their employee morale and job satisfaction.

(59) Which of the following statements regarding professional communication is incorrect?

(A) The current healthcare system has many interfaces and patient handoffs between mental healthcare practitioners.

(B) During a short hospital stay, a patient may interact with fifty different staff members, such as nurses, psychiatrists, and technicians.

(C) Accurate communication of critical information is necessary in an effective clinical practice.

(D) Miscommunication between healthcare providers does not put patients in danger.

(60) Which of the following is considered a chief cause of treatment delays and medication errors?

(A) Communication failures.

(B) Patient's non-compliance.

(C) Insufficient lightning in the hospital room.

(D) The nurse's ethnic background.

(61) What is it called when healthcare providers take on complementary roles, share responsibility, and make decisions when developing a plan for patient care?

(A) Communication.

(B) Cultural Consideration.

(C) Collaboration.

(D) Intervention.

(62) The approach in which all team members from various disciplines work together in an effort to develop a common goal for the patient is called:

(A) Interdisciplinary approach.

(B) Multidisciplinary approach.

(C) Multifaceted approach.

(D) Undivided approach.

(63) Which of the following is not a component of successful teamwork?

(A) A respectful atmosphere and compassionate environment.

(B) A clear decision-making process.

(C) Frequent communication and sharing of information.

(D) Lack of confidence in other team members.

(64) Which of the following is not an obstacle in the development of a collaborative environment?

(A) Loss of autonomy.

(B) Lack of confidence in others.

(C) Clash of perceptions.

(D) Balance of member participation during tasks.

(65) Which of the following is not an example of a communication failure that may result in an adverse clinical outcome?

(A) Members of the same healthcare team have different priorities for patient care.

(B) Patients are unaware of who is in charge of their care.

(C) Healthcare providers have free access to resources.

(D) Patients receive conflicting information from the healthcare staff.

(66) Disruptive behaviors of physicians and nurses can result in collaboration and communication failures. These issues include inappropriate behavior, conflict, confrontation, verbal abuse, physical abuse, and sexual harassment. These concerns have an impact on staff satisfaction and patient outcomes, such as:

(A) Medical errors.

(B) Improved patient safety.

(C) Decreased lengths of hospital stay.

(D) Improved information flow.

(67) A positive outcome of effective communication is:

(A) Improved patient safety.

(B) Increased preventable mortality.

(C) Medication errors.

(D) Compromised patient safety.

(68) The transfer of critical information, authority, and duty of care for patients between different healthcare providers is called:

(A) Professional communication.

(B) Handoff communication.

(C) Transfer communication.

(D) Effective communication.

(69) Which of the following is not a part of the handoff process?

(A) Communication during shift changes.

(B) Communication between different healthcare providers about patient care.

(C) Communication between family members and patients.

(D) Information tools that help healthcare providers communicate about patient care.

(70) Which of the following is not an issue that occurs due to ineffective handoff communication?

(A) Misunderstandings due to a language barrier.

(B) Failure in patient care.

(C) Compromised patient safety.

(D) Medication errors.

(71) Which of the following is an example of a handoff issue that occurs in organizationally complex acute care hospitals?

(A) Patients call the primary nurse too often.

(B) Patients do not disclose sensitive information.

(C) Too many medical students are present in the room.

(D) Physicians have trouble identifying the primary nurse responsible for the patient.

(72) Which of the following is a mistake associated with sign-out sheets in the handoff process?

(A) Unretained information.

(B) Confidentiality issues.

(C) Incomplete documentation.

(D) Misunderstood technical jargon.

(73) Which of the following statements regarding communication differences between nurses and doctors is correct?

(A) Nurses give broad descriptions, while doctors focus on small details of critical information.

(B) Doctors give broad descriptions, while nurses focus on small details of critical information.

(C) Nurses use too much technical jargon, while doctors use simple vocabulary.

(D) Nurses and doctors use simple sentences when communicating with patients.

(74) When the handoff occurs between physicians or between nurses, the handoff is called:

(A) Interdisciplinary.

(B) Intradisciplinary.

(C) Multidisciplinary.

(D) Interfacility.

(75) Which of the following statements regarding the shift-to-shift handoff process is false?

(A) During shift-to-shift handoff, healthcare providers must ensure patient safety by transmitting important patient care information.

(B) The organizational culture of the clinical setting influences the intershift handoff.

(C) In a clinical setting where the staff can communicate and express concerns openly, the culture is one of safety.

(D) The shift-to-shift handoff does not influence patient outcomes.

(76) What is the advantage of a verbal report on the nursing unit?

(A) It encourages efficiency.

(B) It promotes effective management.

(C) It involves the patient.

(D) It provides an educational opportunity for the staff.

(77) What is the advantage of an audiotaped report as a shift-to-shift handoff method?

(A) It provides face-to-face interaction.

(B) It promotes effective management.

(C) It involves the patient.

(D) It allows nurses to repeat the tape to improve their understanding.

(78) Which factor is most likely to contribute to variations in the quality of documentation?

(A) Use of standardized forms.

(B) Nurse's level of experience and training.

(C) Patient's diagnosis.

(D) Availability of electronic health records.

(79) What is the advantage of a written report as a shift-to-shift handoff method?

(A) It involves the patient.

(B) It provides an educational opportunity for the staff.

(C) It allows the review of essential data.

(D) It provides face-to-face interaction.

(80) The benefit of a verbal report conducted at the patient's bedside as a shift-to-shift handoff method is that:

(A) It is not time-consuming.

(B) The offgoing shift can provide patient care while the oncoming shift gets information about the patient.

(C) It does not cause sensory overload.

(D) It allows patient involvement.

(81) Which of the following statements regarding the therapeutic environment is false?

(A) The therapeutic environment should be a place of acceptance, positive regard, and empathetic understanding.

(B) A patient's experience in a therapeutic environment should be beneficial and pleasant.

(C) The therapeutic environment impacts the initial meeting but has little influence on subsequent meetings.

(D) In the therapeutic environment, patients should feel they can verbalize their thoughts freely and express their behaviors and emotions without judgment.

(82) How can a patient's cultural background most effectively be incorporated into their mental health care plan?

(A) Ignoring cultural differences to avoid bias.

(B) Providing the same care regardless of cultural background.

(C) Using culturally relevant communication styles and interventions.

(D) Relying solely on the family's input for cultural considerations.

(83) The principal consideration when creating a therapeutic environment is:

(A) Safety.

(B) Lightning.

(C) The entrance.

(D) Physical space.

(84) The idea that the most effective therapeutic response occurs in a home setting has brought about the creation of:

(A) Outpatient clinics.

(B) Inpatient hospitals.

(C) Rehabilitation centers.

(D) Home-based interventions.

(85) Which of the following populations are not served in a mental healthcare therapeutic environment?

(A) Patients with developmental disabilities.

(B) Patients with wound infections.

(C) Patients with substance use disorder.

(D) Patients with severe and persistent mental illness.

(86) Which of the following statements regarding the therapeutic environment is false?

(A) Some therapeutic environments exist in a traditional context, while others aim for an integrated healthcare approach.

(B) Studies in environmental psychology have helped determine the type of therapeutic environment that is the most beneficial and pleasing for the patients.

(C) The physical and interactive spaces are two factors that need to be considered when creating a therapeutic environment.

(D) Recommendations about the therapeutic environment are not based on science but on the opinions of people who work in interior design and architecture.

(87) What is an effective strategy for promoting mental health awareness and education in primary school settings?

(A) Providing information only to teachers.

(B) Implementing mental health programs only for children with diagnosed disorders.

(C) Integrating mental health education into the general curriculum for all students.

(D) Relying on parents to teach mental health concepts at home.

(88) How can the lack of parking spaces in the therapy building's parking lot affect the patient's emotional state?

(A) It might make patients irritable and angry at the therapist.

(B) It does not affect the patient's emotional state.

(C) It might make patients feel unwelcome or unwanted.

(D) It can make patients anxious.

(89) A specific environment that is carefully structured in a way that keeps patients safe and provides them with the highest number of benefits is called:

(A) Therapeutic alliance.

(B) Therapeutic milieu.

(C) Home-based service.

(D) Therapeutic office.

(90) The therapeutic milieu can be seen in:

(A) Outpatient and inpatient clinics.

(B) Only in hospitals.

(C) In private therapeutic offices.

(D) In various settings such as rehabilitation facilities, outpatient and inpatient clinics, hospitals, private therapeutic offices, and even at home.

(91) Ideally, where should the waiting room and exit area be located?

(A) In the same location.

(B) Next to each other.

(C) Depends on the clinician's preferences.

(D) In different locations.

(92) Which of the following statements regarding the therapeutic environment's waiting area is false?

(A) It is a place where people begin to collect their inner feelings and thoughts.

(B) It should be a place of calmness.

(C) Talking on the phone should be encouraged to increase the patient's comfort.

(D) The noise level should be kept to a minimum.

(93) In the physical space of the therapeutic environment, the size of the room should be:

(A) Very small to make the patient feel safe.

(B) Very big to avoid potential claustrophobic feelings in patients.

(C) A medium-sized, wide room.

(D) Disregarded as it does not influence the therapeutic alliance.

(94) The decorations in the physical space of the therapeutic environment:

(A) Can have symbolic meaning for patients.

(B) Should express the clinician's religious beliefs.

(C) Should express the clinician's personality.

(D) Are not necessary and may cause more harm than good.

(95) Which of the following statements regarding the seating arrangement in the therapeutic environment is correct?

(A) The patient and the therapist should be near each other (around thirty inches).

(B) The patient and the therapist should be far from each other (around eighty inches).

(C) The patient and the therapist should be at an intermediate distance from each other (between forty-eight and sixty inches).

(D) Patients should not have control over the furniture in the room.

(96) Which of the following lightning choices has the most beneficial effect on patients?

(A) Fluorescent lighting.

(B) Natural lighting.

(C) Dim lighting.

(D) White lighting.

(97) Which of the following is the best color choice for the therapy setting?

(A) Green.

(B) White.

(C) Pink.

(D) Neutral.

(98) White-noise machines can be used in the office to:

(A) Increase the patient's ability to focus.

(B) Sedate the patient to make hypnosis easier.

(C) Ensure confidentiality and increase self-disclosure.

(D) Create a pleasant atmosphere and increase comfort.

(99) Which of the following scents is the most appropriate for the therapeutic environment?

(A) Lavender.

(B) Camomille.

(C) A neutral scent.

(D) Peppermint.

(100) Consistency and behavioral expectations can:

(A) Ensure the patient and therapist know what to expect from each other.

(B) Increase the potential for negative transference.

(C) Increase the potential for positive transference.

(D) Increase the potential for negative countertransference.

(101) Which of the following is a facilitating intervention?

(A) Ask closed-ended questions.

(B) Make judgmental statements.

(C) Minimize the patient's concerns.

(D) Acknowledge the patient's emotions.

(102) A patient shares the story about their traumatic abusive relationship with their ex-husband. During the interview, the psychiatric mental health nurse practitioner uses phrases such as "I see," "hmm," "yes," and "go on." Which intervention is she using?

(A) Reinforcement.

(B) Summarizing.

(C) Reflection.

(D) Reassurance.

(103) A sixty-eight-year-old patient who has alcoholism says: "I would stop drinking if my children would visit me more often!" How would the psychiatric mental health nurse practitioner respond if they were using reflection as a facilitating intervention?

(A) You should call your children and tell them to visit you.

(B) Your children are not being very helpful.

(C) If you stop drinking, your children will visit you more often.

(D) So, if your children visit you more, you will have the motivation to stop drinking.

(104) Which of the following is a facilitating intervention?

(A) Summarizing.

(B) Premature interpretation and advice.

(C) Intense questioning.

(D) Minimizing the patient's concerns.

(105) A twenty-three-year-old patient is diagnosed with bipolar disorder type I. She complains that she worries nobody will want to marry her because of her diagnosis. She says that she heard that she might have to be on medication her whole life and that sometimes the disorder is very difficult to treat. To decrease her anxiety, the psychiatric mental health nurse practitioner:

(A) Reassures the patient and motivates her to continue treatment.

(B) Suggests that she might find someone with the same diagnosis as her.

(C) Warns the patient that if she feels this way, the medication might not work.

(D) Accuses the patient of being very difficult.

(106) During a psychiatric interview, the patient tells a joke, and the psychiatric mental health nurse laughs. How will this action affect the interview process?

(A) Obstruct progress because the patient will think the nurse is laughing at them.

(B) Decrease anxiety and add a genuine feeling to the atmosphere of the interview.

(C) Unfocus the patient as they might start joking to gain positive feedback.

(D) Highlight the clinician's unprofessionalism.

(107) Which of the following conditions is Electroconvulsive Therapy most commonly indicated for?

(A) Generalized Anxiety Disorder.

(B) Major Depressive Disorder.

(C) Borderline Personality Disorder.

(D) Post-Traumatic Stress Disorder.

(108) Which of the following is an obstructive intervention?

(A) Silence.

(B) Minimizing patient's concerns.

(C) Reassurance.

(D) Summarizing.

(109) Early on in an interview with a patient who abuses psychoactive substances, the psychiatric mental health nurse practitioner asks the patient questions such as "When did you start using substances?" "How often do you use substances?" What kind of questions are these?

(A) Open-ended questions.

(B) Reflective questions.

(C) Judgmental questions.

(D) Closed-ended questions.

(110) A seventeen-year-old patient who suffers from bulimia nervosa presents to the emergency department. The psychiatric mental health nurse tells her, "You are ruining your body with your behavior. You have to change!" What kind of statement is this?

(A) A judgmental statement.

(B) A compassionate statement.

(C) Constructive criticism.

(D) An empathetic statement.

(111) During an interview, the psychiatric mental health nurse practitioner looks at her watch and yawns excessively. What might these actions communicate to the patient?

(A) Interest in the patient's story.

(B) Actively listening.

(C) Boredom and disinterest.

(D) Encouragement to share sensitive information.

(112) Which statement regarding obstructive interventions is false?

(A) Judgmental interventions stop the patient from being open about sensitive or intimate information.

(B) Closed-ended questions can halt the progression of the patient's story.

(C) Obstructive interventions disrupt the development of a positive provider-patient relationship.

(D) Premature advice can be productive because it leaves more time to discuss other topics during the interview.

(113) What can intense questioning achieve?

(A) It encourages the patient to open up more about their situation.

(B) It can result in the right answer for the patient's situation.

(C) It can make the patient feel as if they are being interrogated.

(D) It helps the clinician understand the patient.

(114) Which of the following patients will benefit the most from motivational interviewing?

(A) A patient being treated for psychoactive substance use but has mixed feelings about change.

(B) A patient with treatment-controlled schizophrenia.

(C) A patient with borderline personality disorder who is diligent in using DBT skills.

(D) A patient with depression who is compliant with their medication.

(115) What is the main purpose of motivational interviewing?

(A) To increase the patient's self-compassion.

(B) To increase the patient's motivation for change by resolving their ambivalence.

(C) To gain as much information about the patient as possible.

(D) To help create the most appropriate treatment plan.

(116) Which of the following core skills of motivational interviewing allows the patient to reflect and elaborate before answering?

(A) Affirmation.

(B) Reflective listening.

(C) Summarizing.

(D) Open-ended questions.

(117) Which of the following core skills of motivational interviewing increases the patient's self-confidence and encourages them to take action?

(A) Affirmation.

(B) Reflective listening.

(C) Summarizing.

(D) Open-ended questions.

(118) A type of reflective listening that consists of repetition or rephrasing of statements is called:

(A) Active listening.

(B) Closed listening.

(C) Simple listening.

(D) Complex listening.

(119) Which of the following best describes complex reflective listening?

(A) Paraphrasing the patient's words without adding any interpretation.

(B) Reflecting the patient's feelings and the underlying meaning behind their words.

(C) Providing direct advice and solutions to the patient's problems.

(D) Asking closed-ended questions to gather specific information.

(120) People who have mental illness in Asian-American communities are:

(A) Provided with mental health support early on.

(B) Not stigmatized by the society.

(C) Understood by their families.

(D) Seen as people with out-of-control behavior.

(121) Which of the following is the largest ethnic minority group in the United States?

(A) African Americans.

(B) Arab Americans.

(C) Latin Americans.

(D) Asian Americans.

(122) The dominant religion in Latin-American communities is:

(A) Roman Catholicism.

(B) Islam.

(C) Protestantism.

(D) Buddhism.

(123) Which of the following populations is known to experience a greater burden of mental illness?

(A) Adolescents.

(B) Older adults.

(C) People living in rural areas.

(D) Low-income individuals.

(124) Which of the following best describes the role of emotional and physical touch?

(A) Always avoid physical touch to maintain professional boundaries.

(B) Physical touch should only be used as a last resort during a crisis.

(C) Emotional support and appropriate physical touch can build trust and rapport.

(D) Emotional and physical touch are not relevant in mental health nursing.

(125) Which of the following statements regarding gender roles in Muslim communities is correct?

(A) Men are expected to be subordinate to women.

(B) There are no traditional gender roles in Muslim societies.

(C) Women are expected to be subordinate to men.

(D) Women take the role of the protector and provider.

(126) Which of the following statements regarding mental illness in the Arabic community is correct?

(A) People with mental illness are provided with mental health support early on.

(B) People with mental illness are not stigmatized by the society.

(C) People with mental illness talk about their issues openly.

(D) People with mental illness tend to present with vague somatic complaints.

(127) What a body does to a drug is defined as:

(A) Pharmacodynamics.

(B) Pharmacokinetics.

(C) Bioavailability.

(D) Dose-response curve.

(128) Which of the following statements is true regarding metabolism in the context of psychotropic medications?

(A) Metabolism of psychotropic medications is solely dependent on the patient's diet.

(B) Metabolism of psychotropic medications is not influenced by genetic factors.

(C) Variations in metabolism can affect the efficacy and side effects of psychotropic medications.

(D) All patients metabolize psychotropic medications at the same rate.

(129) A forty-year-old male patient with schizophrenia is treated with aripiprazole (Abilify). The patient's symptoms are not reacting to the medication. After a careful medication review, the psychiatric mental health nurse practitioner notices that this patient is taking carbamazepine. How does carbamazepine affect the therapeutic effect of aripiprazole?

(A) Carbamazepine is a cytochrome P450 inducer, and aripiprazole is a cytochrome P450 substrate.

(B) Carbamazepine is a cytochrome P450 inhibitor, and aripiprazole is a cytochrome P450 substrate

(C) Carbamazepine is a cytochrome P450 substrate, and aripiprazole is a cytochrome P450 inducer.

(D) Carbamazepine is a cytochrome P450 substrate, and aripiprazole is a cytochrome P450 inhibitor.

(130) A thirty-two-year-old female patient who suffers from depression and insomnia has been on treatment with mirtazapine for the last ten years. In the past weeks, she has reported an increase in adverse effects. After a careful review of her medication, the psychiatric mental health nurse practitioner noticed that a month ago, the patient was diagnosed with peptic ulcer disease and was treated with cimetidine. How does cimetidine affect the therapeutic effect of mirtazapine?

(A) Cimetidine is a cytochrome P450 substrate, and mirtazapine is a cytochrome P450 inhibitor.

(B) Cimetidine is a cytochrome P450 substrate, and mirtazapine is a cytochrome P450 inducer.

(C) Cimetidine is a cytochrome P450 inhibitor, and mirtazapine is a cytochrome P450 inducer.

(D) Cimetidine is a cytochrome P450 inhibitor, and mirtazapine is a cytochrome P450 substrate.

(131) For pharmacokinetics, what does "distribution" refer to?

(A) The process of a drug being absorbed into the bloodstream.

(B) The elimination of a drug from the body.

(C) The dispersion of a drug throughout the body's fluids and tissues.

(D) The chemical transformation of a drug within the body.

(132) When a medication is described as one that exerts an agonistic effect, it means that the medication:

(A) Activates a biological response.

(B) Causes the opposite effect of the agonist by binding to the same receptor.

(C) Partially activates the receptor.

(D) Binds to the receptor without activating it.

(133) Which of the following statements regarding the pharmacological management of psychiatric drugs is false?

(A) Identifying the phase of the illness (acute or chronic phase, relapse or recurrence) has implications for treatment.

(B) A medication review should be done to identify potential interactions between prescribed medications (including non-psychiatric drugs).

(C) Personal and family history of response to medications should be recorded to identify positive or adverse responses.

(D) The clinician has no responsibility to inform the patient about the length of treatment since there is a risk of non-compliance if the patient is aware that it may be an extended period.

(134) A twenty-three-year-old patient with schizophrenia is about to start treatment with a medication that is associated with a serious side effect (agranulocytosis). The psychiatric mental health nurse practitioner should register the medication in the Risk Evaluation and Mitigation Strategies (REMS) database. Which medication has this patient been prescribed?

(A) Olanzapine.

(B) Diazepam.

(C) Clozapine.

(D) Thioridazine.

(135) Medication-induced movement disorders are caused by:

(A) A blockade of serotonin reuptake pumps responsible for the reuptake of serotonin back to the presynaptic neuron.

(B) Antagonism of muscarinic receptors.

(C) Inhibition of the enzyme monoamine oxidase.

(D) Blockade of dopamine type 2 receptors.

(136) A seventy-two-year-old male patient with schizophrenia put on haloperidol develops a tremor of the lips and perioral muscles, drooling, and coarse tremor of the hands on the tenth day of treatment. The psychiatric mental health nurse practitioner should:

(A) Order creatinine phosphatase levels since the patient may be developing neuroleptic malignant syndrome.

(B) Diagnose idiopathic parkinsonism.

(C) Prescribe levodopa.

(D) Treat the patient with benztropine.

(137) A life-threatening complication that may occur during treatment with antipsychotics which presents with muscular rigidity, dystonia, mutism, akinesia, obtundation, agitation, hyperthermia, increased pulse and blood pressure, diaphoresis, an elevated white blood cell count, as well as increased creatinine phosphokinase, plasma myoglobin, liver enzymes, and myoglobinuria on laboratory examination is called:

(A) Serotonin syndrome.

(B) Neuroleptic malignant syndrome.

(C) Tardive dyskinesia.

(D) Medication-induced acute akathisia.

(138) A twenty-one-year-old male patient with a psychotic disorder treated with haloperidol presents with abnormal protrusions of the tongue, trismus, and oculogyric crises. This side effect is called:

(A) Medication-induced acute dystonia.

(B) Medication-induced acute akathisia.

(C) Tardive dyskinesia.

(D) Neuroleptic-induced parkinsonism.

(139) A forty-one-year-old female patient who suffers from major depressive disorder with psychotic features is prescribed treatment with fluoxetine and olanzapine. She complains of feeling a sense of anxiety and being unable to relax. Upon physical examination, the clinician noticed that she performs rocking motions while sitting. The psychiatric mental health nurse practitioner:

(A) Increases the dose of fluoxetine and reduces the dose of olanzapine.

(B) Decreases the dose of fluoxetine and increases the dose of olanzapine.

(C) Reduces the dose of fluoxetine and olanzapine and adds propranolol.

(D) Stops fluoxetine and adds propranolol.

(140) A twenty-three-year-old female patient with schizophrenia has been on treatment with risperidone for the past eight months. She presents with abnormal protruding movements of the tongue and chewing jaw movements. What is this side effect called?

(A) Medication-induced acute akathisia.

(B) Neuroleptic malignant syndrome.

(C) Rabbit syndrome.

(D) Tardive dyskinesia.

(141) Which of the following medications has the least risk of producing tardive dyskinesia?

(A) Olanzapine.

(B) Haloperidol.

(C) Aripiprazole.

(D) Clozapine.

(142) Which of the following side effects is associated with serotonergic agents?

(A) Tardive dyskinesia.

(B) Akathisia.

(C) Gastrointestinal disturbances.

(D) Neuroleptic malignant syndrome.

(143) Which of the following patients' safety can be endangered by SSRI treatment?

(A) A kindergarten teacher.

(B) A taxi driver.

(C) A secretary in a law firm.

(D) A medical doctor.

(144) Which of the following actions is not useful in treating somnolence?

(A) Adjust the dosage of the medication that causes somnolence.

(B) Adjust the timing of administration of the medication that causes somnolence.

(C) Switch to an alternative medication that does not cause somnolence.

(D) Add an SSRI.

(145) The psychiatric mental health nurse practitioner should specifically ask the patient about one side effect caused by SSRIs. Which one?

(A) Sexual dysfunction.

(B) Weight loss.

(C) Gastrointestinal disturbances.

(D) Somnolence.

(146) Which of the following medications can help facilitate weight loss in a patient who is on treatment with Venlafaxine?

(A) Propranolol.

(B) Clopidogrel.

(C) Metformin.

(D) Olanzapine.

(147) Which of the following statements regarding psychoeducational groups is incorrect?

(A) Psychoeducational groups can be practiced in various settings, such as hospitals, universities, or social service agencies.

(B) The leader of a psychoeducational group should have the knowledge, expertise, and skills to guide a wider audience.

(C) Only adults can participate in psychoeducational groups.

(D) Psychoeducational groups can be defined as groups that focus on educating a wide range of audiences on a psychological concept or topic.

(148) What does the KASST model stand for?

(A) Knowledge, Assessment, Skills, Supervision, Training.

(B) Knowledge, Attitudes, Skills, Support, Training.

(C) Knowledge, Application, Skills, Support, Training.

(D) Knowledge, Attitudes, Skills, Supervision, Training.

(149) Since psychoeducational groups deal with various audiences, group leaders should have extensive:

(A) Power.

(B) Knowledge.

(C) Dominance.

(D) Morals.

(150) Which category of the KASST model describes a group leader's process of personal development and self-awareness?

(A) Art.

(B) Science.

(C) Knowledge.

(D) Techniques.

Test 2: Answers and Explanations

(1) (C) Trauma history.

Treatment planning is a complex process that creates a program to provide patients with the most effective treatment. Many different approaches are used to develop a treatment plan. Most share common elements, which include identifying and background information, a list of problems, goals and objectives, intervention strategies and tactics, and flexibility.

(2) (B) Identifying and basic information.

The treatment plan starts with basic information about the patient (e.g., name, age, employment status, and marital status), reasons for starting treatment, and medical and psychiatric history. Information regarding current medical and psychiatric issues, diagnoses, and treatments should also be included.

(3) (D) Referral source and reason for referral.

It is important to identify the individual or organization that referred the patient for treatment and the reason for the referral. Often, patients recognize that they have a problem and seek resources and health providers to help them cope. These patients are self-referred. In some cases, someone aware of the patient's problem makes the referral.

(4) (C) "The patient has been feeling on edge lately. He worries that his wife might leave him because he lost his job. He cannot fall asleep at night. He feels hopeless and lost."

The treatment plan includes the patient's reasons for seeking treatment. The main complaint should be written in the patient's own words. The patient's description can give more detailed information about the issue, its intensity, and its effect on their life compared to the clinician's description. In this case, the clinician might write, "The patient suffers from an anxious-depressive state." However, the patient's description conveys a more complete picture.

(5) (D) The problems should be described generally, e.g., "school problems."

The problems should be written in clear and unambiguous language. The example, "school problems," is not descriptive enough and may have different meanings. Better descriptions include "undisciplined behavior during class," "aggressive behavior toward peers," or "academic underachievement." Precise descriptions enable clinicians to pinpoint the problem that needs to be the focus of the intervention.

(6) (C) Family dynamics.

The family environment, including relationships with parents, siblings, and other significant family members, can significantly influence a person's emotional and psychological development. Understanding family dynamics helps mental health professionals identify patterns of behavior, communication styles, and potential sources of stress or support that may impact the patient's mental health.

(7) (B) Is there a problem that poses a danger to the patient or others?

The first step is to assess if a problem poses a threat to the patient or others. These issues include suicidality, homicidality, domestic violence, substance abuse or dependence, and neglect of children or others in the patient's care.

(8) (A) A problem that, if treated, might destabilize the patient.

A problem that might destabilize the patient is a lower-priority problem that should be addressed later in treatment. Questions that help prioritize problem lists include:

- Is there a problem that poses a danger to the patient or others?
- What problem has the most impact on the patient's life?
- Which problem, if resolved, will solve many or most of the other problems?
- Is there a problem that is easily solvable?

(9) (A) Limitations of a healthcare plan.

Patient factors that constrain the length of treatment include limited healthcare plan benefits, a patient's reluctance to engage in treatment for an extended period, and other potential issues related to the patient. Clinician factors include reduced practice hours, closing the practice, and other clinician-controlled issues.

(10) (D) DSM-V.

The payer of the treatment chooses the diagnostic classification system. The DSM-V is the most commonly used. In some cases, the ICD-10 is required. However, the DSM-V is the most prevalent among healthcare providers. It is the standard taught in residencies, internships, and graduate school courses.

(11) (C) Abstract.

Well-formed goals and objectives should be specific, measurable, achievable, realistic, and time-limited (SMART). Abstract goals do not provide clear guidance or criteria for evaluating progress, which makes them less effective in a treatment plan.

(12) (D) Specific.

Specific goals can be measured. For example, if a person with social anxiety says that their goal is to "feel better," that is a nonspecific goal that would be difficult to measure. If their goal is to have at least one conversation with a stranger per day, that goal is specific and measurable.

(13) (B) Measurable.

A measurable goal can be quantified. This allows a clinician to monitor a patient's progress. The data is used to evaluate if the chosen treatment is effective and helps determine if any adjustments are necessary. Patients can see how much they have progressed since the beginning of treatment, which motivates them to continue actively participating.

(14) (D) It is unachievable in the specified timeline.

Given her circumstances, this patient's goal is unachievable. It is unlikely that the patient will be able to lose twenty pounds in one week, and exercising for three hours every day would be unhealthy and stressful for her body. Clinicians are often faced with patients who want to accomplish unachievable goals. Unachievable goals should be avoided regardless of the pressure third parties might put on the clinician.

(15) (A) Realistic.

Does the patient have enough motivation to put in the required work? Do family members and significant others provide enough support? How will external factors influence the process? Will the patient's insurance company pay for the treatment? The reality of the situation must always be considered since working toward an unrealistic goal results in adverse outcomes.

(16) (C) Time-bound.

A realistic timeline for completing a goal shows that the clinician believes the patient can achieve the goal in a timely fashion. This can increase the patient's self-esteem and motivate them to achieve the set goals and objectives.

(17) (B) The treating clinician.

A clinician uses a treatment plan to guide a patient's progress. It is a tool that enables them to facilitate therapeutic intervention. The clinician will use the treatment plan more than anyone else. In most cases, the clinician who develops the treatment plan is the one responsible for the patient.

(18) (C) The patient.

The patient should agree to the problems identified, the treatment goals and objectives, and the therapeutic interventions. The treatment plan is a source of reassurance for the patient and can hold both patient and clinician accountable for the roles they have agreed to before starting treatment.

(19) (B) Insurers.

Insurers may require the treatment plan to ensure the quality of care or as a formality. The treatment plan conveys information that the health plan member is receiving appropriate and adequate care and provides evidence that the treatment is medically necessary.

(20) (C) Whether the patient is a danger to others.

Third parties are most interested in whether the patient is a danger to others and whether the patient can benefit from treatment; therefore, these issues should be adequately addressed in the treatment plan. Examples of interested third parties include courts, state vocational rehabilitation agencies, law enforcement officers, special education service providers, the military, and the clergy.

(21) (C) The beliefs people have about spirituality.

Cognitive behavioral therapy is based on the cognitive model, which states that people's perceptions and reactions to situations are shaped by cognitive structures, also called schemas. Cognitive structures are people's beliefs about themselves, the world around them, and the future. This is called the cognitive triad. These thoughts are developed by the person's life experiences and depend upon their constitution.

(22) (A) Depression.

CBT is based on the cognitive model, which states that cognitive structures shape people's perceptions and reactions to situations. Negative maladaptive cognitive structures caused by negative emotional experiences are associated with many psychiatric disorders, such as depression, anxiety disorder, panic disorder, personality disorders, obsessive-compulsive disorders, and somatoform disorders. The cognitive theory of depression states that people with depression have a negative view of themselves, a negative view of the future, and a negative interpretation of their experiences.

(23) (D) Help her elicit automatic thoughts and test their validity with cognitive behavioral therapy techniques.

The cognitive distortions described in the question are all-or-nothing thinking and catastrophizing. The therapist should teach the patient to test and carefully examine exaggerated automatic thoughts and generate alternative explanations for events. For example, the patient might be too socially anxious because she feels bad about her physical appearance, so she does not talk to people.

(24) (B) A negative belief about himself.

This patient has a negative belief about himself. He believes he is inadequate and does not deserve his current job. The cognitive theory of depression states that people with depression have a negative view of themselves, a negative view of the future, and a negative interpretation of their experiences. Correcting negative maladaptive cognitive structures can improve the patient's symptoms and condition.

(25) (D) Journal daily activities.

Keeping a journal of daily activities is a behavioral technique used in CBT. Behavioral techniques help change and test maladaptive cognitions to challenge the inaccuracy of a patient's maladaptive cognitive structures while developing new, more adaptive coping methods. Behavioral techniques include journaling, scheduling activities, self-reliance training, cognitive rehearsal, graded task assignments, and diversion techniques.

(26) (B) Teach her to identify and test maladaptive assumptions.

Maladaptive assumptions can guide a patient's life and cause the development of a psychiatric disorder such as depression. A maladaptive assumption in this patient is, "If I am not perfect, nobody will love me." The psychiatric mental health nurse practitioner can help patients identify maladaptive assumptions and test their validity by providing alternative explanations.

(27) (C) Patients with psychiatric diseases do not need additional empowerment.

Many patients with psychiatric diseases may feel helpless and dependent on mental health services. Empowerment can make them feel as if they have more control. It involves autonomy, courage, personal responsibility, and demanding the same rights as other people without a mental illness. Patients' self-sufficiency can be empowered with appropriate income and housing, adequate access to healthcare, and freedom from violence.

(28) (C) A patient with schizophrenia who believes that ghosts are after him.

Psychotic disorders are not an indication for cognitive behavioral therapy. CBT can be used as isolated treatment or combined with medications to:

- Reduce psychological distress or symptoms of a mental illness.
- Change beliefs that enable the development of disorders.
- Draw attention to psychosocial factors.
- Minimize the chance of relapse after remission has occurred.
- Increase compliance with treatment.

(29) (B) Dialectical Behavior Therapy.

Dialectical Behavior Therapy is specifically designed to help individuals with borderline personality disorder improve their interpersonal relationships, emotional regulation, and distress tolerance skills. DBT combines cognitive-behavioral techniques with mindfulness practices to address the complex needs of these patients.

(30) (C) Supportive psychotherapy.

Supportive psychotherapy can be used to treat all mental disorders, such as psychoses and dementia. Supportive psychotherapy is individual psychotherapy used to help patients through difficult times and situations. Patients can discuss any problems they experience, which may range from issues in their marriage to persecutory delusions caused by psychosis. The therapist should express concern, sympathy, and interest.

(31) (A) Help patients through difficult times and situations.

Supportive psychotherapy is individual psychotherapy used to help patients through difficult times and situations. Patients can discuss any problems they experience, which may range from issues in their marriage to persecutory delusions caused by psychosis. The therapist should express concern, sympathy, and interest.

(32) (B) Specific coping techniques.

Therapists teach patients specific coping techniques, such as how to learn new skills, incorporate new hobbies in their daily routine, meet new people, or achieve autonomy. Alcoholic patients who have stopped drinking may receive words of encouragement and suggestions on how to increase self-control and how to spend their free time, for example, playing new sports or developing creative hobbies.

(33) (D) It requires therapists to undergo extensive psychotherapy.

Group therapy provides patients with a safe and secure environment where they can share their problems, reduce feelings of loneliness and isolation, and learn new coping skills. It can also help patients improve their social skills. Inpatient groups are usually followed by outpatient or after-care groups. These groups are used to follow up with patients and consolidate the skills they have learned in the inpatient setting.

(34) (C) Trauma-informed care.

Individuals who experience trauma and stress can negatively engage with healthcare services. There is a chance of re-traumatization when a trauma survivor interacts within the healthcare system. Trauma-informed care enables healthcare providers to understand the impact of trauma on their patients and adapt to the needs of trauma survivors to improve clinical outcomes.

(35) (C) An open and non-threatening body position.

Patients with a history of trauma might be reminded of past experiences when they interact with a provider with a threatening body posture. This may trigger feelings of powerlessness. Providers should be aware of their body language and use non-threatening body positions to help patients stay regulated.

(36) (B) Ask the patient for permission every time before measuring their blood pressure.

Physical touch can be associated with unpleasant traumatic memories; therefore, it can activate the fight, flight, or freeze response in trauma survivors. The psychiatric mental health nurse practitioner should ask for permission before touching patients, even after performing a task multiple times in a day (e.g., when measuring a patient's blood pressure).

(37) (D) Ask the medical students to leave the room.

Patients have the right to privacy. They should be able to choose the people physically present during their care. If there are people in the room that the patient feels uncomfortable with (e.g., medical students), the nurse should ask them to leave. The responsibility of asking others to leave should not be put on the patient since they may not feel empowered to do so.

(38) (C) "Hi. I know we have met before, but I would like to remind you that I am your mental health nurse and will take care of you during your stay."

The psychiatric mental health nurse practitioner should introduce themselves and their role in every interaction. Patients interact with many medical staff members during their care, and because of this, they may not remember each person's function. Clinicians should reiterate their role to prevent confusion.

(39) (C) Patients should not be informed what to expect since that might cause too much anxiety.

The medical staff should provide anticipatory guidance and tell the patient what to expect. For example, they should inform them that they will have several laboratory tests today or visits from the resident doctors. Patients with trauma are not comfortable with surprises since past trauma may have been unpredictable. Informing them of the healthcare plan will make them feel more in control and regulated.

(40) (A) Self-identity.

Having a mental illness can damage one's sense of self. Re-developing the lost sense of self is a significant part of the recovery journey. The illness, as it is only a part of the self, should be considered separately. The patient can re-establish their identity and develop self-respect as they accept and grieve what was lost and gain a healthy understanding of their experience.

(41) (D) Lack of side-effects.

Patients may choose complementary interventions for reasons such as a desire for more control in the decision-making process, low insurance coverage for conventional treatment, a preference for natural health alternatives, and side effects and failure of medications.

(42) (B) Complementary interventions.

Complementary interventions are defined as non-conventional treatments that are added to conventional medical treatment. Alternative interventions are defined as non-conventional treatments that are given instead of conventional medical treatment. Integrative methods combine both conventional and non-conventional treatments. Complementary interventions can be categorized into natural, biologically based treatments (e.g., vitamins, supplements, herbal products, and aromatherapy), mind and body interventions, and whole systems and body-based therapies (e.g., massage, Ayurvedic medicine, reflexology).

(43) (B) Explain that omega-3 is not an effective monotherapy for depression but can be used in combination with an antidepressant.

Docosahexaenoic acid (DHA) is an omega-3 polyunsaturated fatty acid. It can be used for attention deficiency disorder, dyslexia, cognitive impairment, and dementia. It can also be useful as a complementary medicine for patients with depression who are on a conventional antidepressant. However, it is not useful as a monotherapy for depression. The psychiatric mental health nurse practitioner should explain that the benefits of an antidepressant outweigh the potential side effects.

(44) (C) Explains to the patient that he should not take Choline due to his genetic condition.

Choline can be used in patients with manic conditions, tardive dyskinesia, cancer, and cognitive disorders. It is needed for the structure and function of all cells and is beneficial for fetal brain development. The dosage is 300-1200 mg, but higher doses (above three grams) are associated with a fishy body odor. Adverse effects include sweating, hypotension, and depression. Choline should be restricted in patients with primary genetic trimethylaminuria.

(45) (A) Immediately discontinues both fluoxetine and 5-HTP.

This patient may be presenting with serotonin syndrome since he is taking two serotonergic agents. 5-HTP is an immediate precursor of serotonin. It is useful in depression, obesity, fibromyalgia, and headaches. Patients with carcinoid tumors or those who take MAOIs have a risk of serotonin syndrome with 5-HTP. 5-HTP interacts with SSRIs, MAOIs, methyldopa, St. John's wort, phenoxybenzamine, 5-HT antagonists, and 5-HT receptor agonists.

(46) (A) Vitamin E.

Vitamin E can increase a patient's risk of bleeding, hemorrhagic stroke, and thrombophlebitis. Vitamin E interacts with warfarin, antiplatelet drugs (e.g., aspirin), and neomycin. Due to the increased risk of bleeding, vitamin E should be stopped prior to surgical procedures.

(47) (D) Vitamin E.

Vitamin E is in the essential fat-soluble vitamin family, which is made of tocopherols and tocotrienols. It has immune-enhancing, antioxidant, and neuroprotective properties. It is used in neurologic disorders, diabetes, and premenstrual syndrome. It may alleviate symptoms of depression, irritability, and weight gain in patients with PMS.

(48) (C) Melatonin.

Melatonin occurs naturally in the body. It is a hormone produced by the pineal gland that regulates the circadian rhythm and sleep. It can be used for insomnia, sleep disturbances, and jet lag. Adverse effects of melatonin include seizures, grogginess, depression, headache, and amnesia. It can also inhibit ovulation in higher doses (more than 1 g)

(49) (B) Sertraline and St. John's wort.

St. John's wort (*Hypericum*) is effective for the treatment of major depressive disorders, anxiety, and sleep problems. It contains hypericin, flavonoids, and xanthones. Adverse effects include headaches, photosensitivity, and constipation. St. John's wort should not be used with SSRIs or MAOIs. There is a risk of serotonin syndrome and reports of mania when combined with sertraline (Zoloft). It should not be used with alcohol or opioids.

(50) (C) Valerian.

Valerian (*L.Valeriana officinalis*) contains valepotriates, valerenic acid, and caffeic acid. It is used as a sedative, muscle relaxant, and hypnotic. Valerian can cause cognitive and motor impairment, gastrointestinal upset, and hepatotoxicity. Long-term use is associated with contact allergy, headaches, restlessness, insomnia, mydriasis, and cardiac dysfunction.

(51) (D) Gingko.

Gingko (*L. Gingko biloba*) contains flavonoids and ginkgolides. The benefits of gingko include symptomatic relief of delirium and dementia, as well as improved concentration and memory. Gingko is a possible antidote to sexual dysfunction caused by SSRIs. Adverse effects include allergic skin reactions, gastrointestinal upset, muscle spasms, and headaches. Gingko has potential interactions with anticoagulants and increases the risk of bleeding.

(52) (A) Ginseng.

Ginseng (*L.Panax ginseng*) contains triterpenes and ginsenosides. Ginseng has stimulating and mood-elevating properties. It can cause insomnia, hypertonia, and edema (also called ginseng abuse syndrome). Ginseng should not be used with sedatives, hypnotic agents, MAOIs, antidiabetic agents, or steroids. Due to its anticoagulant action, it should be discontinued seven days before surgery.

(53) (D) Kava kava.

Kava kava is used as a sedative, hypnotic, and antispasmodic. It can cause lethargy, impaired cognition, and dermatitis in patients who use it long-term. Kava kava is synergistic with anxiolytics and alcohol. Kava kava should be avoided in patients who are treated with levodopa and other dopaminergic agents. It is contraindicated in patients with endogenous depression since it can increase the danger of suicide.

(54) (B) Lavender.

Lavender (*L. Lavandula angustifolia)* contains hydroxycoumarin, tannins, and caffeic acid. It is used for its sedative and hypnotic properties. Essential oils from lavender are used in aromatherapy to treat anxiety. Adverse effects include headache, nausea, and confusion. Lavender is synergistic with other sedatives. The dosage is three to five grams per day, and an overdose can cause death.

(55) (C) A forty-five-year-old patient with schizophrenia who has his illness under control with 4 mg risperidone.

Patients who benefit the most from natural products or supplements are those who prefer natural products, have too many intolerable adverse effects from medications, or have inadequate nutrient intake. Products that should be considered are evidence-based, have logical mechanisms of action, a high benefit-to-risk ratio, and have a defined dosage and time frame that allows for evaluating their effects.

(56) (B) Lorazepam.

Lorazepam is a benzodiazepine commonly used to treat anxiety disorders. One of the primary side effects of benzodiazepines, including lorazepam, is somnolence, or excessive drowsiness. This occurs because benzodiazepines enhance the effect of the neurotransmitter gamma-aminobutyric acid (GABA) at the GABA-A receptor, which has a calming effect on the brain, often leading to sedation and drowsiness.

(57) (B) Care coordination.

Care coordination is a process necessary to help patients with mental health issues receive the best possible care and achieve the best outcome. It can be defined as the deliberate organization of patient care activities between healthcare professionals. Healthcare providers interact with clinicians, patients, family members, caretakers, and other important persons. The coordination of services can help ensure that the patient receives the proper treatment at the right time.

(58) (A) Receive the right services at the right time.

Care coordination's main goal is to ensure that every patient receives the appropriate services and support at the right time. The focus is on providing close communication and collaboration between various healthcare professionals, such as mental health providers, psychiatrists, psychologists, primary care providers, psychiatric mental health nurse practitioners, social workers, and community mental health centers.

(59) (D) Miscommunication between healthcare providers does not endanger patients.

Miscommunications between healthcare providers can endanger patient safety due to misinterpretation, lack of critical information, unclear orders, and unnoticed changes in the patient's physical or psychiatric status. Healthcare providers have various levels of education and occupational training. A patient may interact with fifty different staff members, such as nurses, psychiatrists, and technicians, during a short hospital stay. All employees must have close collaboration.

(60) (A) Communication failures.

Lack of communication can cause medical errors, which can result in injury or patient death. Communication failures are considered among the principal causes of delays in treatment and medication errors. Clear communication and collaboration between team members are necessary to minimize the rate of medical errors and ensure patient safety.

(61) (C) Collaboration.

Collaboration in healthcare is achieved when healthcare providers work together cooperatively. They take on complementary roles, share responsibility, and make decisions that aid in the development of patient care plans. By collaborating, healthcare team members gain awareness of each other's skills and knowledge, which improves decision-making. Respect, collaboration, and trust characterize the most effective teams.

(62) (A) Interdisciplinary approach.

An interdisciplinary approach should be implemented in healthcare for a successful teamwork model. In a multidisciplinary approach, every team member takes responsibility for actions related to their own discipline and develops separate goals for the patient. In an interdisciplinary approach, all team members from various disciplines work in a joint effort to develop a common goal for the patient.

(63) (D) Lack of confidence in other team members.

A lack of confidence in others does not result in successful teamwork. The most important components of successful teamwork include a clear direction, open communication, well-defined roles for the members, a respectful atmosphere and compassionate environment, a balance of member participation during tasks, a straightforward decision-making process, an enabling environment, accessible resources, frequent communication and sharing of information, conflict resolution skills, and appropriate mechanisms for outcome measurement and ability to adjust accordingly.

(64) (D) Balance of member participation during tasks.

The balance of member participation during tasks is not an obstacle to developing a collaborative environment. Obstacles include a perceived loss of autonomy, a clash of perceptions, additional time, and a lack of confidence in others. These obstacles can be overcome by fostering mutual respect and trust and keeping an open attitude. Collaboration and teamwork are among the most important factors to improve clinical effectiveness.

(65) (C) Healthcare providers have free access to resources.

Communication failures that result in adverse clinical outcomes can sometimes be attributed to social and relational structures. Members of the same healthcare team can have different priorities for patient care, which may cause inconsistencies in verbal communication. Many patients have reported that during their hospital stay, they were unaware of who was in charge of their care, and the healthcare staff provided them with conflicting information.

(66) (A) Medical errors.

Communication failures can result in adverse patient outcomes such as medical errors, preventable mortality, adverse effects, and patient risk. Many healthcare professionals have gotten used to communication and teamwork failures, which have developed into a culture of low expectations in the healthcare setting. In this type of culture, many medical errors can occur because even the most diligent healthcare providers start to ignore discrepancies and red flags and expect a partial and faulty exchange of information.

(67) (A) Improved patient safety.

It is important to remember that effective communication can result in many positive outcomes, such as effective therapeutic interventions, improved patient safety, improved patient and family satisfaction, decreased length of hospital stay, enhanced job satisfaction and employee morale, and improved information flow. Effective communication encourages continuous and clear patient care, fosters teamwork, and minimizes medical errors.

(68) (B) Handoff communication.

Handoff communication is the transfer of critical information, authority, and duty of care for the patient between different healthcare providers. An effective handoff consists of a continuous and effective transition of essential information, care, and treatment.

Inadequate handoff communication results in adverse outcomes and compromised patient safety. Other terms related to handoff include cross-coverage, shift report, and sign-out.

(69) (C) Communication between family members and patients.

Communication between family members and patients is not part of the handoff process. Handoff is a complex process that involves the transfer of critical information, authority, and duty of care for the patient between different healthcare providers. The process ensures that essential information about the patient is conveyed successfully.

(70) (A) Misunderstandings due to a language barrier.

With the specialization and evolution of healthcare, the number of providers in patient care has increased. Because of this, there are more handoffs in the current healthcare delivery system compared to the less complex systems in the past. Issues of handoff can result in failure of patient care, compromised patient safety, medication errors, and increased morbidity and mortality. There are many challenges for effective communication in the complex and dynamic clinical setting.

(71) (D) Physicians have trouble identifying the primary nurse responsible for the patient.

The complex organization and increased number of specialties and physicians that provide care to one patient contribute to difficulties in communication in organizationally complex acute care hospitals. Many physicians have reported that they are often unable to identify the patient's primary nurse, and many nurses have had trouble identifying the patient's primary physician.

(72) (C) Incomplete documentation.

An example of an ineffective handoff is the use of sign-out sheets. Doctors frequently use sign-out sheets for communication. However, they are associated with incomplete documentation, such as missing allergies, weight, and errors in medication information.

(73) (A) Nurses give broad descriptions, while doctors focus on small details of critical information.

Doctors and nurses communicate differently. Nurses tend to focus on the big picture and give broad descriptions of situations, while physicians often concentrate on smaller details of critical information. The SBAR (situation, background, assessment, recommendation) briefing model is one technique that aims to improve handoff communication by bridging the communication style gap between doctors and nurses.

(74) (B) Intradisciplinary.

The handoff is called interdisciplinary when the transfer occurs between nurses and physicians or nurses and diagnostic personnel. When the handoff occurs between physicians or between nurses, it is called intradisciplinary. When handoffs occur between hospitals and organizations such as extended-care facilities or home health agencies, the handoffs are called interfacility handoffs.

(75) (D) The shift-to-shift handoff does not influence patient outcomes.

The shift-to-shift handoff is a complex process, which, if done poorly, may result in adverse patient outcomes. Many human factors influence this process during shift changes. During shift-to-shift handoff, healthcare providers must transmit important patient care information, promote continuous patient care, and confirm that the patient is transferred to a competent and qualified nurse to ensure patient safety. The organizational culture of the clinical setting influences the intershift handoff. In a setting where the staff can communicate and express concerns openly, the culture is one of safety.

(76) (D) It provides an educational opportunity for the staff.

A verbal report on the nursing unit can provide an educational opportunity for the staff and allow face-to-face interactions. It can help clarify information and allow time to debrief and discuss situations. The downside is that the receiver may not retain information because the report is verbal only, which can be time-consuming and cause sensory overload. An augmented verbal report with preprinted forms that contain data about the specific patient can reduce the loss of information.

(77) (D) It allows nurses to repeat the tape to improve their understanding.

An audiotaped report is more efficient, concise, and repeatable. Nurses can replay the tape to understand the information better. As the nurses from the oncoming shift listen to the audiotaped report, the nurses who taped it can provide patient care. The sound quality of the recording should be ensured to improve the audiotaped report.

(78) (B) Nurse's level of experience and training.

The nurse's level of experience and training significantly impacts the quality of documentation. Experienced and well-trained nurses are more likely to provide thorough, accurate, and consistent documentation, which is necessary for effective patient care and communication among healthcare providers.

(79) (C) It allows the review of essential data.

A written report allows the oncoming shift to review essential data. It will enable effective management and improve documentation. However, a written report may have weaknesses due to variations in the quality of documentation and the absence of question-and-answer interaction. A standardized process should be used to ensure that essential information is conveyed.

(80) (D) It allows patient involvement.

A verbal report at the patient's bedside has certain strengths, such as patient involvement, face-to-face interaction, and the ability to clarify information. However, it has confidentiality issues and issues related to the use of technical jargon, which may concern the patient if not properly explained. Clinicians can introduce the nurses, encourage patients to participate, monitor to ensure protected confidentiality, and use a developed protocol that will guide the handover process to overcome these issues.

(81) (C) The therapeutic environment impacts the initial meeting but has little influence on subsequent meetings.

When a patient enters the hospital or any other space, the environment is the first thing they encounter. The therapeutic environment will affect how the person experiences the initial and subsequent meetings. It should be a place of acceptance, positive regard, and empathetic understanding. In the therapeutic environment, patients should feel they can verbalize their thoughts freely and express their behaviors and emotions without judgment.

(82) (C) Using culturally relevant communication styles and interventions.

Incorporating a patient's cultural background into their mental health care plan involves using communication styles and interventions that are culturally relevant.

(83) (A) Safety.

Safety is the first priority when creating a therapeutic environment. A simple way to assess safety is for a clinician to ask themselves whether they feel safe working in the environment. If they do not feel safe, they can ask themselves, what can they do to increase their sense of safety?

(84) (D) Home-based interventions.

Psychology has played a role in shaping the spaces used for therapeutic purposes. The idea that the most effective therapeutic response occurs in a home setting has resulted in the creation of intensive in-home and other home-based interventions. These services are delivered in the patient's home, which means the therapist does not control the process.

(85) (B) Patients with wound infections.

The most commonly served populations in the therapeutic environment include patients with severe and persistent mental illness, developmental disabilities, and substance use disorder. They can be treated in different locations and receive a variety of services specific to their needs. These patients can be helped through residential programs, outpatient programs, or day programs.

(86) (D) Recommendations about the therapeutic environment are not based on science but on the opinions of people who work in interior design and architecture.

Studies in environmental psychology have helped determine the type of therapeutic environment that is the most beneficial and pleasing for patients. These studies have used surveys that ask people whether they have felt comfortable where they have received therapy. Many factors come into play when discussing the structure of the environment. Therapy can be done in clinics, community spaces, facilities, homes, private practice offices, counseling centers, rehabilitation centers, and other community-based locations.

(87) (C) Integrating mental health education into the general curriculum for all students.

Integrating mental health education into the general curriculum ensures that all students receive information and resources about mental health. This promotes early awareness, reduces stigma, and equips children with the knowledge and skills to manage their mental well-being effectively.

(88) (C) It might make patients feel unwelcome or unwanted.

The size of the parking lot should be considered, and spaces for vehicles used by people with disabilities must be included. There should be enough parking spaces for all patients coming to therapy since a lack of parking spaces can make people feel unwanted or unwelcome. There should also be enough parking spaces for staff and visitors.

(89) (B) Therapeutic milieu.

The therapeutic milieu is a carefully structured, specific environment that keeps patients safe and provides them with the highest number of benefits. Milieu therapy enables patients to learn new skills and encourages positive attitudes such as respect and positivity. It supports patients on the journey toward recovery. Patients who trust in the therapeutic milieu feel empowered to try new adaptive coping skills.

(90) (D) In a variety of settings such as rehabilitation facilities, outpatient and inpatient clinics, hospitals, private therapeutic offices, and even at home.

The therapeutic milieu is seen in various settings such as rehabilitation facilities, outpatient and inpatient clinics, hospitals, private therapeutic offices, and even at home. Milieu therapy is not limited to a safe physical environment but includes supportive therapists, nurses, and other healthcare staff. Milieu therapy consists of a structured environment, support, consistent expectation, mutual respect, a focus on the needs of the patient, evenly distributed power, and repetition.

(91) (D) In different locations.

The interactions between people when they exit the building should be considered. If possible, the exit and waiting area should be in different locations. The entrance should be free from obstruction so people can locate the waiting area. The receptionist should be pleasant and warm. There should be a private space to collect confidential data. The entrance should be made accessible for patients with disabilities.

(92) (C) Talking on the phone should be encouraged to increase the patient's comfort.

The waiting area is a place to step away from the stress of daily life into the calmness of a counseling session. It is where people gather their inner feelings and thoughts. Therefore, the noise level should be minimal. Phone use should be discouraged since people might not want to overhear conversations.

(93) (C) A medium-sized, wide room.

A small room can negatively influence therapeutic communication, while a wide room can support a healthy therapeutic alliance. However, if the room is too big, it may elicit feelings of insecurity in the patient. A pleasant and well-maintained physical space should make people feel comfortable. To increase self-disclosure, the room where therapy is conducted should be a warm and intimate setting.

(94) (A) Can have a symbolic meaning for patients.

Office decorations can have symbolic meanings for patients. Clinicians should consider that decorations can induce a particular belief, which may cause negative or positive transference. Plants are a positive decoration since they remind patients of natural environments. Pictures of nature can also have a calming effect.

(95) (C) The patient and the therapist should be at an intermediate distance from each other (between forty-eight and sixty inches).

The patient and therapist should be between forty-eight and sixty inches apart. People feel a sense of autonomy and increased comfort when they can control movable furniture, like chairs or pillows. Adults should sit in large chairs or sofas, while children should be in small chairs.

(96) (B) Natural lighting.

Natural lighting has the most beneficial effect on patients. It reduces negative emotions and increases self-disclosure. However, if natural lighting is not possible, use dim or soft lighting instead of fluorescent lighting. These options have a calming effect on patients. Lamps and indirect lighting make the atmosphere more pleasant.

(97) (D) Neutral.

Preferences for color vary across different ages and genders. However, neutral, soft, and light colors are the most practical choices for a therapy setting. This choice can elicit a sense of calmness for both the patient and the therapist.

(98) (C) Ensure confidentiality and increase self-disclosure.

White noise machines can make the patient more comfortable with self-disclosure, as they ensure confidentiality. The healthcare staff should minimize external and office noise so the therapeutic session is not interrupted. Patients feel more comfortable fully engaging in therapy when they are in soundproof rooms.

(99) (C) A neutral scent.

Scents can trigger old memories and emotional or physical responses. Therefore, the office should have a neutral smell and no intense perfumes or colognes. Soft textures create a comfortable setting. The ideal temperature is between sixty-eight and seventy-two degrees Fahrenheit (average room temperature). Patients may become distracted if they feel too hot or too cold.

(100) (A) Ensure the patient and therapist know what to expect from each other.

Establishing expectations, consistency, and boundaries can create a safe environment. It should feel homelike to the patient, who should be able to express themselves without expecting or fearing rejection. By providing consistency and behavioral expectations, the patient and therapist will know what to expect from each other.

(101) (D) Acknowledge the patient's emotions.

Patients share feelings more openly when their emotions are acknowledged. They feel relieved if they know they can candidly express their thoughts. Nonverbal actions such as putting the tissue box closer to the patient can be helpful if used appropriately. If the patient is clearly expressing an emotion, it is better to comment on the associated feelings rather than directly commenting on the emotion.

(102) (A) Reinforcement.

Reinforcement might seem like a simple technique, but it is a very useful method that encourages patients to share more information about their situation. Reinforcement uses simple phrases such as "I see," "hmm," "yes," and "go on." These phrases show that the interviewer is interested and motivates the patient to continue talking. They should fit naturally into the interview.

(103) (D) So, if your children visit you more, you will have the motivation to stop drinking.

Reflection uses the patient's words. It informs the patient that the clinician is listening, they understand, and they want to know more. Reflections should be said in a challenging tone. To avoid sounding robotic, paraphrase the patient's words.

(104) (A) Summarizing.

Summarizing should be done during the interview. It sums up what has been discussed. By summarizing, psychiatrists can share their understanding of the situation. The patient can clarify or add new information if needed. The psychiatrist might use the information to expand the discussion or explore the new information later.

(105) (A) Reassures the patient and motivates her to continue treatment.

The psychiatric mental health nurse practitioner can reassure the patient by presenting her with factual information about the outcomes of bipolar disorder type I and motivate her to continue her treatment to improve her outcomes. Reassuring the patient is helpful because it can decrease their anxiety about the illness and encourage them to continue the discussion about the illness. When there are many unknown variables, the nurse can provide reassurance that they are always available and willing to help however they can.

(106) (B) Decrease anxiety and add a genuine feeling to the atmosphere of the interview.

Sometimes, patients like to tell jokes. Smiling or laughing at the joke can be helpful in this situation since sharing humor decreases anxiety and adds a genuine feeling to the atmosphere of the interview. The clinician should be sure that the patient intended to make a funny comment and that they are laughing at the joke, not the patient.

(107) (B) Major Depressive Disorder.

Electroconvulsive Therapy is most commonly indicated for Major Depressive Disorder, particularly in cases where the patient has not responded to other treatments such as medication and psychotherapy. ECT is also used in patients who require a rapid response due to severe symptoms, such as those experiencing suicidal ideation or catatonia. The procedure involves the application of controlled electric currents to the brain, which can quickly alleviate severe depressive symptoms.

(108) (B) Minimizing patient's concerns.

Sometimes, the therapist minimizes the patient's concern in an attempt to reassure them. In this situation, the patient might feel that the therapist does not truly understand their suffering. Exploring the concern can result in the discovery of new information that may be relevant to the treatment plan.

(109) (D) Closed-ended questions.

Closed-ended questions can halt the progression of the patient's story. Patients can come prepared for therapy, especially if they have previous experience. They are ready to talk about painful topics. If the psychiatrist blocks the patient by asking too many closed-ended questions, the patient cannot be a partner in the interview. Psychiatrists learn to refine their skills during the interview.

(110) (A) A judgmental statement.

Judgmental statements prevent patients from being open about sensitive or intimate information. They are nonproductive and can obstruct the development of a respectful relationship. Criticizing, disagreeing, and blaming can make the patient feel something is wrong with them. Sometimes, patients can interpret a simple disagreement as critical. It may be more beneficial to ask the patient if they think their actions result in productive results.

(111) (C) Boredom and disinterest.

The importance of nonverbal communication should not be underestimated. A therapist who checks their watch, yawns, looks at a computer screen, or turns away from the patient may seem disinterested or bored. These actions could make a patient feel unimportant, which could ruin the relationship between the provider and the patient.

(112) (D) Premature advice can be productive because it leaves more time to discuss other topics during the interview.

When a therapist makes premature interpretations, a patient might feel misunderstood and act defensively, even when the interpretation is correct. Premature advice is counterproductive because, early in the interview, the therapist does not know all the factors at play. This might obstruct the patient's wish to create a plan.

(113) (C) It can make the patient feel as if they are being interrogated.

Intense questioning can be mistaken for good listening. A clinician might want to ask more questions to get to know the patient better, but this might make the patient feel as if they are being interrogated. Often, asking too many questions does not result in the right answer.

(114) (A) A patient being treated for psychoactive substance use but has mixed feelings about change.

Motivational interviewing is helpful for patients who are treated for psychoactive substance abuse, smoking cessation, reduction of HIV-risk behaviors, eating disorders, and poor medication compliance. It is also beneficial for patients who are ambivalent (mixed feelings about change), have low self-confidence (doubt they can change), have a low desire to change, or are unaware of the advantages of change.

(115) (B) To increase the patient's motivation for change by resolving their ambivalence.

Motivational interviewing is a client-centered method that aims to increase patients' motivation for change by resolving their ambivalence. It meets patients at the level of their problem recognition. Patients may respond better to a family-centered model that uses motivational interviewing rather than the disciplinary expert-providing advice approach.

(116) (D) Open-ended questions.

Open-ended questions enable patients to tell their stories, compared to closed-ended questions used to gather brief information. They allow patients to reflect and elaborate before answering. Their answers will help the clinician understand things from their perspective. Open-ended questions start dialogues and do not require a specific answer from the patient.

(117) (A) Affirmation.

Affirmation expresses positive regard and genuine appreciation for a patient. When affirming, highlight the patient's past successes, strengths, and efforts. The statements should emphasize the patient's accomplishments using "you" instead of "I." For example, rather than, "I am happy you came in here today," say, "You are working hard to improve your life and make a positive change."

(118) (C) Simple listening.

Reflective listening requires the healthcare provider to actively listen to the patient, hypothesize the meaning or emotion of their statement, and reflect the best interpretation back to them. Simple reflective listening, which consists of repeating or rephrasing statements, is less challenging than complex reflections.

(119) (B) Reflecting the patient's feelings and the underlying meaning behind their words.

Complex reflective listening involves not only repeating what the patient has said but also interpreting and reflecting back the underlying emotions and meanings. This helps to deepen the patient's self-awareness and shows empathy.

(120) (D) Seen as people with out-of-control behavior.

Psychiatric illness is often seen as out-of-control behavior in Asian-American communities. There is great shame for individuals who have a mental illness. Families attempt to manage them on their own until it gets impossible to handle. Many individuals may present with somatic complaints when suffering from mental distress since it is seen as more acceptable than expressing genuine emotions.

(121) (C) Latin Americans.

Latin Americans comprise the largest ethnic minority group in the United States. They trace their ancestry throughout the Americas and beyond, in countries such as Puerto Rico, Cuba, Spain, and Mexico. Spanish is the common language, and it has many dialects. Latinos use a lot of touch in their communication and appear agreeable and diplomatic. They are group-oriented people who prefer to interact with large groups of relatives.

(122) (A) Roman Catholicism.

The dominant religion in the Latin-American community is Roman Catholicism. Religion has a strong influence on their lives, and this influence increases during times of crisis. Roman Catholicism and Spanish and Indian ideologies influence the folk beliefs of health. The male folk healer is called the curandero, and the female folk healer is called the curandera. Traditional Latin Americans believe that folk healers have a gift from God that allows them to heal the sick.

(123) (D) Low-income individuals.

Low-income individuals experience a greater burden of mental illness due to factors such as increased stress, lack of access to healthcare, social determinants of health, and limited resources for support and treatment.

(124) (C) Emotional support and appropriate physical touch can build trust and rapport.

Emotional support and appropriate physical touch, when used correctly, can help build trust and rapport between the nurse and the patient. It can convey empathy, provide comfort, and support therapeutic relationships.

(125) (C) Women are expected to be subordinate to men.

Arabic families have defined gender roles. Men are the head of the household and are considered protectors and decision-makers. Women are subordinate to men and are responsible for caring for children and fulfilling their husbands' needs. The main social organization is the family, and loyalty to the family is considered more important than one's personal needs. Women's modesty is valued.

(126) (D) People with mental illness tend to present with vague somatic complaints.

There is much stigma around mental illness in the Arabic community. People believe that psychiatric symptoms are due to the presence of "evil spirits" or "bad nerves." Many people who suffer from mental distress present with vague somatic complaints such as shortness of breath, abdominal pain, or anorexia.

(127) (B) Pharmacokinetics.

Pharmacokinetics is defined as *what a body does to a drug*. It refers to the movement of a drug in, through, and out of a body. A patient's response to a drug depends on genetic and environmental factors. Drugs that are effective in some patients may not be effective in others. Drugs differ from each other in their molecular structure, interactions with neurotransmitters, pharmacokinetics, protein binding, and the presence of active metabolites. Drug and patient factors influence treatment efficacy, tolerability, and safety.

(128) (C) Variations in metabolism can affect the efficacy and side effects of psychotropic medications.

Variations in metabolism are influenced by genetic factors and other variables, and they can significantly impact how effectively psychotropic medications work and the side effects experienced by patients.

(129) (A) Carbamazepine is a cytochrome P450 inducer, and aripiprazole is a cytochrome P450 substrate.

First-pass metabolism refers to the metabolization of drugs by the cytochrome P450 enzymes in the liver and intestines before reaching systemic circulation. Cytochrome P450 inducers increase the metabolism and decrease the therapeutic concentration of drugs. They include carbamazepine, St. John's wort, phenytoin, phenobarbital, and tobacco. Carbamazepine increases the metabolism of aripiprazole and, therefore, decreases its therapeutic concentration, which is why the patient is not seeing benefits from his treatment.

(130) (D) Cimetidine is a cytochrome P450 inhibitor, and mirtazapine is a cytochrome P450 substrate.

First-pass metabolism refers to the metabolization of drugs by the cytochrome P450 enzymes in the liver and intestines before reaching systemic circulation. Cytochrome P450 inhibitors decrease the metabolism and increase the therapeutic concentration of the drugs. They include bupropion, clomipramine, cimetidine, clarithromycin, fluoroquinolones, grapefruit, ketoconazole, nefazodone, and SSRIs. Cimetidine decreases the metabolism of mirtazapine and increases its therapeutic concentration, which is why the patient has experienced more adverse effects since starting cimetidine.

(131) (C) The dispersion of a drug throughout the body's fluids and tissues.

Distribution refers to the way a drug is spread throughout the body's fluids and tissues after it enters the bloodstream. This process determines the concentration of the drug in various parts of the body and affects its efficacy and side effects.

(132) (A) Activates a biological response.

Receptors are the target sites for drugs. When drugs bind to a receptor, they can exert the following.

- Agonistic effects: Activate a biological response.
- Inverse agonistic effects: Cause the opposite effect of the agonist by binding to the same receptor.
- Partial agonistic effects: Partially activate the receptors.

- Antagonistic effects: Bind to the receptor without activating it.

(133) (D) The clinician has no responsibility to inform the patient about the length of treatment since there is a risk of non-compliance if the patient is aware that it may be an extended period.

The psychiatric mental health nurse practitioner should inform the patient of the risks and benefits of a treatment and document informed consent. The patient should understand the target symptoms, benefits, adverse effects, risks, potential comorbid complications, and potential alternatives to treatment. Patients should be informed that certain illnesses, such as bipolar disorder, schizophrenia, anxiety disorders, and refractory depression, may require lifelong treatment.

(134) (C) Clozapine.

Clozapine is an antipsychotic that is associated with the development of agranulocytosis, which is a serious side effect. Treatment with clozapine should be registered in the Risk Evaluation and Mitigation Strategies (REMS) database. Other serious side effects with medical consequences include hepatic failure (nefazodone), heart block (thioridazine), stroke (phenelzine), and Stevens-Johnson syndrome (lamotrigine). Drugs that carry a risk of life-threatening consequences must be closely monitored.

(135) (D) Blockade of dopamine type 2 receptors.

Medication-induced movement disorders are most commonly associated with drugs used to treat psychosis (DRAs) and second-generation antipsychotics (SGAs). The mechanism behind the abnormal motor activity is the blockade of dopamine type 2 (D2) receptors. Since SGAs block dopamine receptors to a lesser extent than first-generation antipsychotics, they are less likely to cause movement disorders.

(136) (D) Treat the patient with benztropine.

This patient is presenting with neuroleptic-induced parkinsonism, and therefore, he should be treated with an anticholinergic agent such as benztropine. Signs and symptoms include muscle stiffness (lead pipe rigidity), cogwheel rigidity, stooped posture, drooling, coarse tremors, tremors of the lips and perioral muscles (rabbit syndrome), and shuffling gait. Parkinsonian side effects usually occur five to ninety days after starting treatment and most commonly affect elderly and female patients.

(137) (B) Neuroleptic malignant syndrome.

Neuroleptic malignant syndrome is a rare, potentially life-threatening complication that may occur during treatment with antipsychotics. The symptoms can last from ten to fourteen days if left untreated. The diagnosis can be missed since the withdrawal or increased agitation may mimic the exacerbation of psychosis. Treatment includes supportive medical treatment and medications such as dantrolene, bromocriptine, and amantadine. The antipsychotic dose should be as low as possible. High-potency drugs have the highest risk of inducing neuroleptic-malignant syndrome.

(138) (A) Medication-induced acute dystonia.

Dystonia is defined as prolonged muscle contractions that cause abnormal movements or postures. It can present as oculogyric crises, tongue protrusions, trismus, laryngeal-pharyngeal dystonias, dystonic postures of the limbs and trunk, trismus, blepharospasm, and glossopharyngeal dystonia. Dystonia most commonly affects men, patients younger than thirty, and patients who are on high-potency antipsychotics.

(139) (C) Reduces the dose of fluoxetine and olanzapine and adds propranolol.

This patient complains of akathisia, a subjective feeling of restlessness, or objective visible signs of restlessness associated with antipsychotic, sympathomimetic, and antidepressant treatment. Patients complain of a sense of anxiety and inability to relax. On examination, they present with jitteriness, rocking motions while sitting, pacing back and forth, and alterations between sitting and standing. Treatment consists of reduction of the medication to the lowest effective dose possible and beta-adrenergic receptor antagonists.

(140) (D) Tardive dyskinesia.

Tardive dyskinesia is a late-appearing side effect of antipsychotics. The patient presents with abnormal involuntary movements that affect the head, extremities, and trunk muscles with variable severity. The most commonly affected area is the perioral area, which includes twisting and protruding tongue movements, lip-puckering, grimaces of the face, and chewing and lateral jaw movements.

(141) (D) Clozapine.

Clozapine has the least risk of tardive dyskinesia and may even be used to improve symptoms due to its low D2 receptor affinity and high 5-HT receptor antagonism. The development of tardive dyskinesia can be prevented by using antipsychotics in the lowest effective doses only when indicated. SGAs are associated with less tardive dyskinesia.

(142) (C) Gastrointestinal disturbances.

Older antidepressants and antipsychotics have significant gastrointestinal side effects, such as constipation, due to their anticholinergic activity. Newer drugs act on the serotonin system and have very little anticholinergic activity. Since the majority of serotonin is located in the gastrointestinal tract, serotonergic medication can be a cause of abdominal pain, nausea, diarrhea, and flatulence.

(143) (B) A taxi driver.

SSRIs may cause somnolence due to impaired sleep quality. Somnolence may impair patients' quality of life and endanger the safety of those who operate vehicles (e.g., a taxi driver) or any type of mechanical equipment. Patients who are on chronic treatment with SSRIs may experience fatigue or exhaustion despite getting adequate amounts of sleep.

(144) (D) Add an SSRI.

SSRIs may cause somnolence due to impaired sleep quality. Patients who are on chronic treatment with SSRIs may experience fatigue or exhaustion despite getting adequate amounts of sleep. Somnolence can be managed by adjusting the dosage or the timing of administration. Another option is to add small doses of stimulants or modafinil. The clinician can also consider switching to an alternative medication that does not cause somnolence.

(145) (A) Sexual dysfunction.

Sexual dysfunction caused by SSRIs consists of decreased libido, inability to orgasm, and impaired ejaculation and erection. Even though sexual dysfunction is amongst the more common side effects, patients often do not report it spontaneously. Therefore, asking the patient specifically about this side effect is important.

(146) (C) Metformin.

Olanzapine and valproate cause insulin resistance, which increases appetite and, therefore, increases weight. Metformin can make weight loss possible in patients who gain weight because of treatment with serotonin-dopamine reuptake inhibitors and valproic acid.

(147) (C) Only adults can participate in psychoeducational groups.

Psychoeducational groups can include children, adolescents, and adults. They can be practiced in various settings, such as hospitals, universities, or social service agencies. The leaders of these groups provide guidance for personal learning, show members how to decrease isolation and help each other, foster hope, promote self-awareness, find opportunities for new learning, and create a safe space for emotional expression.

(148) (D) Knowledge, Attitudes, Skills, Supervision, Training.

The KASST model stands for Knowledge, Attitudes, Skills, Supervision, and Training. This model emphasizes the comprehensive development of a nurse's capabilities in mental health care.

(149) (B) Knowledge.

Since psychoeducational groups deal with various audiences, group leaders should have extensive knowledge about the groups and their focuses. This is necessary in order to teach effectively. Group leaders need to understand group dynamics, stages of development, therapeutic factors, processes, ethics, instructional principles, and conditions or topics.

(150) (A) Art.

The art of the group depends on the group leader's self-awareness and personal development. The authentic self of the group leader manifests through their expression of warmth, tolerance, respect, caring, and genuineness. Group members can sense the authenticity of the group leader without them verbalizing it. Personal development impacts many aspects, such as cultural sensitivity, countertransference, and unconscious negative impact. Group leaders are encouraged to be introspective and work on potentially unresolved issues.

Test 3: Questions

(1) What is the goal of mental health promotion?

(A) Change people's maladaptive cognitive patterns.

(B) Improve cognitive restructuring.

(C) Increase awareness about medication management.

(D) Develop positive mental health for individuals with mental health problems and the community in general.

(2) Which of the following is the main goal of disease management?

(A) Reducing hospital readmissions.

(B) Increasing patient dependence on medication.

(C) Minimizing contact with healthcare providers.

(D) Encouraging isolation from social support networks.

(3) Mental health promotion advocates for whose emotional and social well-being?

(A) People with substance use disorders.

(B) People with neurological disease.

(C) People that are without, at risk of, or with mental illness.

(D) People without mental illness.

(4) Which of the following is not a goal of mental health promotion?

(A) Relapse prevention.

(B) Improving coping skills of communities in the face of adversity.

(C) Enabling healthy workplaces.

(D) Increasing tolerance of different cultural backgrounds.

(5) Interventions conducted before the onset of mental illness to prevent its development are called what?

(A) Mental health promotion.

(B) Mental health prevention.

(C) Mental health literacy.

(D) Mental health awareness.

(6) What is the goal of primary mental health prevention?

(A) Reduce or delay the recurrence, frequency, and interval of psychiatric disorders.

(B) Shorten the time a patient spends with a psychiatric disorder.

(C) Lessen the distress, pain, and suffering associated with a psychiatric disorder.

(D) Minimize the incidence and prevalence of certain psychiatric disorders.

(7) What is the goal of relapse prevention?

(A) Prevent or reduce the recurrence of a disorder and the exacerbation of symptoms.

(B) Minimize the distress, pain, and suffering associated with a psychiatric disorder.

(C) Reduce the incidence and prevalence of certain psychiatric disorders.

(D) Limit risk factors of social and environmental conditions, and high-risk behaviors associated with psychiatric disorders.

(8) Which of the following is not a component of a successful relapse prevention plan?

(A) Increased awareness.

(B) Policy changes, social action, and economic management.

(C) Identification of triggers and warning signs.

(D) Mutual collaboration between staff.

(9) Which of the following statements is false regarding resilience?

(A) Patients differ in their ability to cope with adverse situations and avoid breaking down when confronted with stressful events.

(B) Coping and defensive mechanisms can be healthy or maladaptive.

(C) Resilience depends only on the patient's constitution.

(D) Protective factors are not always visible and may become detectable when the person is faced with a stressor.

(10) When should risk factors that predispose individuals to mental illness be identified?

(A) At the end of treatment.

(B) When measuring the outcome.

(C) Early in the mental health assessment process.

(D) During the course of treatment.

(11) Which of the following is not a risk factor for mental illness?

(A) Poor or interrupted development or maturity.

(B) Family discord.

(C) A positive temperament.

(D) Lack of social support.

(12) Incorporating the development of protective factors when caring for patients can help them achieve a higher level of functioning, prevent recurrence of their illness, decrease psychiatric disability and social isolation, develop coping skills, and promote optimum recovery. Which of the following can be used to promote protective factors in the community?

(A) Anti-bullying programs in schools.

(B) Identification of risk factors.

(C) Screening for tobacco use.

(D) Emotionally focused therapy (EFT).

(13) Which of the following is not a protective factor against mental illness?

(A) Emotional intelligence.

(B) Reliable friendships.

(C) Poor nutrition.

(D) Social belonging.

(14) Which of the following antidepressant medications is used to aid tobacco cessation?

(A) Sertraline.

(B) Fluoxetine.

(C) Mirtazapine.

(D) Buproprion.

(15) What is best for patients who are addicted to nicotine when they are admitted to the hospital?

(A) Not allow them to smoke and recommend they use this situation to stop smoking completely.

(B) Avoid interference with their habit.

(C) Provide them with nicotine-replacement therapy.

(D) Remind them about the negative impact of smoking at every encounter.

(16) Who should the psychiatric mental health nurse practitioner assess for tobacco use?

(A) Patients who look like they are smokers.

(B) Every patient who is admitted.

(C) Young children and adolescents.

(D) Assessment for tobacco use is not part of the initial assessment.

(17) Which coping mechanism is most effective for managing extreme stress that comes with mental health disorders?

(A) Avoidance.

(B) Suppression.

(C) Problem-focused coping.

(D) Emotional numbing.

(18) How long should patients be advised to exercise?

(A) At least 120 minutes every day.

(B) At least 60 minutes every day.

(C) At least 30 minutes every day.

(D) Only if they feel like exercising.

(19) Which of the following is not beneficial for patient self-care?

(A) Adherence to a regular sleeping schedule.

(B) Minimal exposure to blue light before bed.

(C) Use an app for meditation.

(D) Watch TV shows before bed.

(20) Which of the following people should seek professional help?

(A) A person who has forgotten to water their plants for the past two days.

(B) A person who had a bad night's sleep the night before.

(C) A person who has been eating poorly for the past month and has unexpectedly lost six pounds.

(D) A person who did not get out of bed because of sadness for two days.

(21) Which of the following scenarios is not an emergency situation?

(A) A 23-year-old female patient who was sexually abused by her male best friend.

(B) A 40-year-old male patient with bipolar disorder who is in the depressive phase and is expressing suicidal thoughts.

(C) A 45-year year old female patient without mental illness who comes to the hospital in a state of massive anxiety because her husband is threatening to kill her and their children.

(D) A 34-year-old male patient who comes to the hospital for the first time because he is having trouble falling asleep for the past month.

(22) Which of the following statements is false regarding the emergency psychiatry treatment setting?

(A) The setting in which the emergency psychiatric evaluation is done must have an atmosphere of safety and security.

(B) The emergency team should be educated and trained in the proper practice of restraints.

(C) Medical conditions do not present with emergency psychiatric manifestations.

(D) Patients who present with physical or emotional distress are in a vulnerable position.

(23) Which of the following scenarios may require abandoning the usual rules of confidentiality?

(A) A 20-year-old female patient with PTSD who is talking about the impact of childhood sexual abuse by a relative on her life.

(B) A 34-year-old male patient with major depressive disorder reports that he is planning to kill himself because life is not worth living.

(C) A 55-year-old female patient with schizophrenia is talking about the voices that are telling her that she is the most incompetent person in the world.

(D) A 28-year-old male patient with OCD reports that they must wash their hands exactly fifteen times before having breakfast.

(24) A 45-year-old male patient with schizophrenia comes in the emergency psychiatry department yelling that he will fight anyone who tries to come near him. The psychiatric mental health nurse practitioner should do what in this case?

(A) Administer IM haloperidol.

(B) Administer IV diazepam.

(C) Physically restrain the patient.

(D) Talk to him in a calm voice and say, “You will not harm anyone.”

(25) Which of the following signs is not typical for an emergency psychiatric condition with a medical etiology?

(A) Acute onset in a patient with comorbid medical illness.

(B) Visual hallucinations.

(C) Disorientation and neurologic signs.

(D) Young age at onset.

(26) Which of the following medical conditions can cause mental status changes that resemble mental illness?

(A) Uncomplicated cystitis.

(B) Diabetic ketoacidosis.

(C) Mild anemia.

(D) Hypertension.

(27) Discovering the underlying reason behind violent behavior has implications for the choice of interventions. Which of the following personality disorders has the highest likelihood of being associated with violent behavior?

(A) Antisocial Personality Disorder.

(B) Borderline Personality Disorder.

(C) Avoidant Personality Disorder.

(D) Schizoid Personality Disorder.

(28) Which of the following signs is not an alert of impending violence?

(A) Psychomotor retardation.

(B) Alcohol intoxication.

(C) Persecutory ideation in a psychotic patient.

(D) Catatonic excitement.

(29) During the interview, the clinician should make a differential diagnosis of violent behavior and attempt to predict the risk of violence. Which of the following patients is at most risk of conducting a violent act?

(A) An elderly female patient with dementia who has persecutory delusions and hallucinations.

(B) A teenage male student with anxiety whose parents are going through a divorce.

(C) A homeless 28-year-old male patient with a substance abuse problem.

(D) A 45-year-old female patient with narcissistic personality disorder.

(30) A state of tension or restlessness that can result in purposeless and disorganized violent behavior is called what?

(A) Agitation.

(B) Catatonia.

(C) Aggression.

(D) Paranoid ideation.

(31) Which of the following methods is the first-line treatment for agitated patients?

(A) Benzodiazepines.

(B) Antipsychotics.

(C) Physical restraints.

(D) Verbal de-escalation.

(32) When should the psychiatric-mental health nurse practitioner ask if the patient has thoughts of suicide?

(A) When the patient is suffering from a mood disorder.

(B) When the patient looks depressed.

(C) When the patient expresses feelings of hopelessness.

(D) Every patient should be asked if they have thoughts of suicide.

(33) Which of the following is not a sign that indicates an increased risk of suicide?

(A) A history of suicidal attempt(s).

(B) History of suicidal ideation.

(C) The presence of an anxiety disorder.

(D) Verbalized suicidal ideation.

(34) A 40-year-old male patient admits that they plan to commit suicide and he is worried how that will affect his wife. What is the best course of action in order to protect this patient's safety?

(A) Hospitalize the patient and have him monitored 24/7.

(B) Send him home and insist that he contact you if the suicidal pressure increases.

(C) Prescribe an antidepressant and discharge him from the hospital.

(D) Hospitalize the patient only if he agrees to be hospitalized.

(35) Which of the following statements is false regarding treating patients with suicidal ideation?

(A) If the patient is not hospitalized, the clinician should insist that the patient contact their healthcare team if suicidal ideation increases.

(B) In the inpatient setting, you must make sure that the patient does not have access to any means by which they can harm themselves, such as glass or other sharp items.

(C) As with any patient who presents with a psychiatric emergency, ensuring safety is a priority.

(D) The nurse should not perform a physical examination on a patient who presents with suicidal ideation since that might make them extremely uncomfortable.

(36) An 18-year-old patient with borderline personality disorder is in crisis. The patient complains of increased suicidal pressure and has had four suicide attempts in her life. Which of the following tests should you order?

(A) Toxicology screen.

(B) Abdominal ultrasound.

(C) Tumor marker levels.

(D) Thyroid function tests.

(37) Which of the following factors does not increase the likelihood of a suicide attempt in the near future?

(A) Use of ethanol.

(B) Access to guns.

(C) Recent suicide attempts.

(D) Grandiose delusions.

(38) Which of the following statements regarding rape and sexual abuse is false?

(A) Rape is often a life-threatening experience since victims are almost always threatened with physical harm.

(B) Rape includes sexual intercourse, anal intercourse, and fellatio.

(C) Rape victims are never male.

(D) The category most at risk of rape is females between the ages of sixteen and twenty-four.

(39) Which of the following medications is most appropriate for a violent, agitated patient who has overdosed on a drug that has anticholinergic properties?

(A) Olanzapine.

(B) Haloperidol.

(C) Diazepam.

(D) Quetiapine.

(40) Which of the following medications is appropriate for a violent patient?

(A) 5 to 10 mg Diazepam slowly and intravenously.

(B) 20 mg Fluoxetine given orally.

(C) 50 mg Clozapine given orally.

(D) 25 mg Sertraline given orally.

(41) Which of the following is the best method to evaluate the effectiveness of treatment?

(A) Patient self-reporting.

(B) Regular clinical assessments.

(C) Medication adherence.

(D) Family feedback.

(42) Choosing inappropriate level of care can cause what?

(A) A breach of confidentiality.

(B) A stagnation of the patient's condition.

(C) An improvement in the patient's condition.

(D) A strong doctor-patient relationship.

(43) The most appropriate type of psychotherapeutic approach for a patient with marital problems is what?

(A) Conjoined marital therapy.

(B) Group therapy.

(C) Individual therapy.

(D) Cognitive therapy.

(44) A patient who has a problem connecting with others will benefit the most from which type of therapy?

(A) Individual.

(B) Group.

(C) Marital.

(D) Cognitive.

(45) Which of the following patients is not a good candidate for psychopharmacologic therapy?

(A) A patient with major depressive disorder.

(B) A patient with schizophrenia.

(C) A patient with marital problems.

(D) A patient with attention-deficit/hyperactivity disorder.

(46) Which of the following patients is a good candidate for psychopharmacologic therapy?

(A) A patient with major depressive disorder.

(B) A patient with marital problems.

(C) A patient with self-esteem issues.

(D) A patient with poor time-management skills.

(47) Which of the following patients is a good candidate for psychopharmacologic therapy?

(A)A patient with major depressive disorder.

(B)A patient with marital problems.

(C)A patient with self-esteem issues.

(D)A patient with poor time-management skills.

(48) Which of the following statements is false regarding treatment effectiveness?

(A) Highly focused treatments are more effective than treatments with a wide focus.

(B) Treatments with a wide focus are more effective than highly focused treatments.

(C) Specific therapy techniques influence treatment effectiveness.

(D) Patient's circumstances and environment influence treatment effectiveness.

(49) The clinician's clinical expertise does not include which of the following?

(A) Diagnostic competence.

(B) Ability to monitor progress.

(C) Ethnic background.

(D) Ability to incorporate new knowledge and skills.

(50) Which of the following is a general consideration that should be implemented before choosing a specific intervention?

(A) Cultural consideration.

(B) Appropriate level of care.

(C) Psychotherapeutic intervention.

(D) Psychopharmacologic intervention.

(51) The expectations that patients have from the clinician's behavior are called what?

(A) Therapist preferences.

(B) Role preferences.

(C) Treatment preferences.

(D) Practice preferences.

(52) The preferences related to the clinician's characteristics are called what?

(A) Practice preferences.

(B) Role preferences.

(C) Therapist preferences.

(D) Treatment preferences.

(53) The preferences related to the specific type of intervention that the patient is expecting to receive are called what?

(A) Treatment preferences.

(B) Therapist preferences.

(C) Practice preferences.

(D) Role preferences.

(54) When a clinician who has a duty to care for patients does something they should not do or does not do something they should do, that is defined as what?

(A) Inattention.

(B) Negligence.

(C) Standard medical practice.

(D) Inconvenience.

(55) In order to prove medical malpractice, the plaintiff (e.g., the patient or their family) should obtain evidence that indicates what?

(A) The patient experienced a side effect from the medication.

(B) The doctor had an arrogant attitude.

(C) The patient got the wrong diagnosis.

(D) The patient was damaged because of a deviation from the standard of care.

(56) In which of the following cases can the psychiatrist be sued for malpractice?

(A) When the psychiatrist prescribes an antidepressant that did not result in a desired outcome.

(B) When the psychiatrist gives advice on television that harms a patient.

(C) When the psychiatrist wrongly diagnoses a patient with OCD.

(D) When the psychiatrist prescribes a medication that is not indicated for the patient's disorder and the patient's condition worsens as a consequence.

(57) Which of the following is not a reason to sue for malpractice?

(A) Intentional tort.

(B) A bad outcome of the patient's condition.

(C) Intentional infliction of emotional distress.

(D) False imprisonment.

(58) Which of the following is not considered a negligent prescription practice?

(A) When a clinician exceeds the recommended doses.

(B) When a clinician mixes medication unreasonably.

(C) When a clinician uses a drug-interaction checker before prescribing medication.

(D) When a clinician prescribes too many medications at the same time.

(59) Which of the following statements is false regarding information when prescribing medication?

(A) The prescribing clinician has no responsibility to give detailed information about the medications they are prescribing.

(B) The prescribing clinician should explain to the patient the diagnosis for which they are receiving medication.

(C) The prescribing clinician should explain the risks and benefits of the proposed treatment.

(D) The prescribing clinician should inform the patient of possible alternatives to the treatment.

(60) When should the clinician obtain inform consent?

(A) Only at the beginning of treatment.

(B) At every follow-up.

(C) At the end of treatment.

(D) After every medication change.

(61) Why is a follow-up interval of one month usually recommended for patients who are receiving treatment?

(A) To minimize the cost of treatment.

(B) To ensure medication compliance and monitor side effects.

(C) To reduce the frequency of patient visits.

(D) To provide patients with more autonomy.

(62) When a psychiatrist prescribes medication and another nonmedical therapist provides psychotherapy, that is called what?

(A)Double treatment.

(B) Joined treatment.

(C) Split treatment.

(D) Collaborative treatment.

(63) What is a key consideration when caring for a secluded patient in a psychiatric setting?

(A) Ensuring they have access to electronic devices.

(B) Providing continuous monitoring for safety.

(C) Allowing them to dictate their own seclusion duration.

(D) Limiting their access to food and water.

(64) Under which circumstance can a psychiatric patient's visitation rights be restricted?

(A) If the patient is sleeping.

(B) If the patient requests no visitors.

(C) If the patient's condition poses a risk to themselves or others.

(D) If the patient does not have any family members.

(65) Which of the following patients should not be allowed unrestricted access to the phone?

(A) A patient who has criminal charges of threatening phone calls.

(B) A patient who has criminal charges of stealing people's belongings.

(C) A patient who is threatening suicide.

(D) A patient who has reduced cognitive abilities.

(66) Which of the following patients should not be secluded except if they are under close supervision?

(A) A patient with antisocial personality disorder and a medical illness.

(B) An 18-year-old patient who has criminal charges of statutory rape.

(C) A 56-year-old agitated schizophrenic patient.

(D) A 67-year-old delirious patient with dementia.

(67) In which of the following scenarios is the doctor released from the responsibility to obtain informed consent?

(A) When a patient is emotionally unstable.

(B) When a patient is being verbally abusive towards the doctor.

(C) When a patient is having a panic attack.

(D) When a mentally incompetent patient is in an emergency situation.

(68) Who provides consent when the patient is legally determined to be mentally incompetent?

(A) Their legal guardian.

(B) The primary care physician.

(C) The psychiatric mental-health nurse practitioner.

(D) A close relative.

(69) Which of the following is not a cause for practicing therapeutic privilege?

(A) Information about the treatment may be too upsetting for the patient.

(B) Information about the treatment might cause a placebo effect.

(C) Information about the treatment might cause severe psychological harm.

(D) Information about the treatment may complicate or obstruct treatment.

(70) Under what condition can a patient be temporarily hospitalized in a psychiatric facility?

(A) If the patient feels lonely.

(B) If the patient needs immediate psychiatric treatment.

(C) If the patient requests it.

(D) If the patient has a minor physical illness.

(71) Which of the following patients cannot be involuntarily hospitalized?

(A) A schizophrenic patient who is aware that he is hearing voices.

(B) A patient who is a danger to himself.

(C) A patient who is unable to take care of his basic personal needs.

(D) A patient who is a danger to others.

(72) When a patient who is involuntarily hospitalized asks that their case be brought before a judge, what happens if the judge decides that the patient should not be hospitalized?

(A) The patient will be released if their psychiatrist agrees with the judge's decision.

(B) The patient will be released if two doctors examine him and agree with the judge's decision.

(C) The patient will be released.

(D) The patient will be released if their family agrees with the judge's decision.

(73) Libel can be defined as:

(A) Written information that damages a person's reputation.

(B) Orally shared information that damages a person's reputation.

(C) An act that makes a person afraid of being touched without consent.

(D) Nonconsensual touching of a person.

(74) The framework and support of the group which includes activities for planning, organizing, structuring, directing, and evaluating is under which category of the KASST model?

(A) Art.

(B) Science.

(C) Knowledge.

(D) Techniques.

(75) Activities that can help promote learning, retention, and participant involvement are under which category of the KASST model?

(A) Art.

(B) Skills.

(C) Science.

(D) Techniques.

(76) The art factors of group leadership cannot be learned since they depend on the individual development of the group leader. How can the personal development of the group leader impact the group?

(A) It can prevent burnout and countertransference.

(B) It can reduce narcissism in other members.

(C) It can make over-participating members self-aware about their behavior.

(D) It can make some group members jealous if they haven't reached their own personal development goals.

(77) When individual thoughts, feelings, and wishes are transferred from a group member to the group leader, the process is called what?

(A) Verbigeration.

(B) Transference.

(C) Countertransference.

(D) Perseveration.

(78) A group member is complaining because his sister is taking their stuff without asking. The group leader starts getting angry because their sister is currently sick in the hospital and the doctors are giving her a bad prognosis. Instead of validating the member's feelings, the group leader says that the group member should be happy they have a healthy sibling in the first place. What is this process called?

(A) Transference.

(B) Countertransference.

(C) Self-Absorption.

(D) Attachment.

(79) Which of the following best describes avoidant behavior for patients with anxiety disorders?

(A) Seeking social interactions to alleviate stress.

(B) Engaging in risky behaviors to feel a sense of control.

(C) Avoiding situations that cause anxiety.

(D) Over-preparing for stressful events.

(80) Which of the following is not a characteristic that the group leader must have?

(A) Confidence in the group.

(B) Ability to accept criticism from others.

(C) Organization skills.

(D) Extreme professionalism without a sense of humor.

(81) How can the group leader effectively understand the group as a whole?

(A) By learning about substance abuse.

(B) By learning about motivation to learn.

(C) By reading books about self-help.

(D) By learning about the group process and group dynamics.

(82) The process of the group that includes the level of participation, resistance, relationship between members and between members and the leader, communication patterns, nonverbal behaviors, feelings expressed, and nonverbal behaviors are called what?

(A) Group stages.

(B) Leadership skills.

(C) Group dynamics.

(D) Helpful group factors.

(83) The level of participation in the group is described by what?

(A) The cooperation and interaction between members and the leader.

(B) The confidence the members have in the leader.

(C) The usefulness of the activities practiced in the group.

(D) Nonverbal communication.

(84) The member who frequently interrupts other members while they are speaking, engages in distracting behaviors, and monopolizes the attention of the group leader is known as what?

(A) Over-participating member.

(B) Under-participating member.

(C) Socializing member.

(D) Disengaged member.

(85) The members who tend to engage in conversations while other members are talking, frequently interact with the same people, introduce different topics while something else is being discussed are known as what?

(A) Under-participating members.

(B) Socializing members.

(C) Over-participating members.

(D) Disengaged members.

(86) The members who are withdrawn, silent, and often make very few responses even when asked a direct question are known as what?

(A) Under-participating members.

(B) Socializing members.

(C) Over-participating members.

(D) Disengaged members.

(87) The member who frequently asks rhetorical questions and tends to zone out during sessions is known as what?

(A) Under-participating member.

(B) Socializing member.

(C) Disengaged member.

(D) Over-participating member.

(88) You can encourage communication between group members by doing what?

(A) Forcefully make them communicate with each other.

(B) Incorporate punishments if members do not talk to each other.

(C) End the session if there is no communication between group members.

(D) Ask members to talk to each other directly.

(89) What does the "feeling tone" of a therapeutic group refer to?

(A) The group's overall emotional atmosphere.

(B) The physical setting of the group meetings.

(C) The specific topics discussed in the group.

(D) The frequency of group sessions.

(90) Why is it important for a mental health nurse to get to know the group members individually?

(A) To provide individualized attention during group sessions.

(B) To control the topics of discussion.

(C) To ensure the sessions run on time.

(D) To monitor the attendance of each member.

(91) If the whole group starts showing resistance, the best course of action is to do which of the following?

(A) Move on to another topic.

(B) Try to break down the resistance.

(C) Start a discussion about the usefulness of the activity.

(D) Terminate the session prematurely.

(92) Which of the following statements regarding psychiatric rating scales is false?

(A) Psychiatric rating scales can be used to monitor the patient's progress over time.

(B) Psychiatric rating scales can be used in research.

(C) Psychiatric rating scales exist only in the format of questionnaires.

(D) Insurers might require psychiatric rating scales to assess the quality of care.

(93) The main purpose of psychiatric rating scales is to do what?

(A) Establish a diagnosis.

(B) Standardize information about the patient which has been collected by various providers.

(C) Assess if the patient has insight about their condition.

(D) Assess if the patient has judgment about their condition.

(94) Which of the following is not achieved with the use of psychiatric rating scales?

(A) Identify any potential comorbid conditions.

(B) Assess factors that impact treatment response.

(C) Predict whether the patient will experience any side effects in response to medication.

(D) Thoroughly describe symptoms.

(95) The broad ranges of areas that scales assess are referred to as what?

(A) Elements.

(B) Features.

(C) Characteristics.

(D) Constructs.

(96) A construct that is used to describe whether a feature is currently present or absent is called what?

(A) Categorical.

(B) Quantitative.

(C) Continuous.

(D) Measuring.

(97) A construct that provides a quantitative assessment of severity, frequency, or intensity is called what?

(A) Categorical.

(B) Continuous.

(C) Classifying.

(D) Dividing.

(98) Which of the following applies to a fully structured formal interview?

(A) The exact wordings of the questions that are asked are specified.

(B) Only some of the wording is specified and additional questions or statements are allowed.

(C) The patient is allowed to add questions to the questionnaire.

(D) Multiple people are interviewing the patient.

(99) Who can administer psychiatric rating scales?

(A) Doctors and nurses.

(B) Doctors, researchers, nurses, social workers, or lay people depending on the type of scale.

(C) Nurses, social workers, or lay people depending on the type of scale.

(D) Doctoral-level clinicians only.

(100) In which of the following scenarios does the clinician need to obtain information from another informant (e.g., a family member) when administering a psychiatric rating scale?

(A) A patient who is in a depressive episode.

(B) A patient who has a panic disorder.

(C) A patient with bipolar disorder currently in remission.

(D) A patient with bipolar disorder currently in a manic episode.

(101) In which of the following scenarios does the clinician not require the use of another informant (e.g., a family member) when administering a psychiatric measuring instrument?

(A) A 73-year-old patient with advanced dementia.

(B) A 54-year-old patient in delirium.

(C) A 60-year-old patient in a depressive episode.

(D) A 7-year-old patient with attention-deficit/hyperactivity disorder (ADHD).

(102) Which is the most commonly used scale to assess disability?

(A) WHO Disability Assessment Schedule scale (WHODAS).

(B) WHO Disability Assessment Schedule scale 2.0 (WHODAS 2.0).

(C) Glasgow Coma Score (GCS).

(D) Disability Ratings Scale (DRS).

(103) Which of the following scales is the gold standard for assessing clinical outcome in studies of schizophrenia treatment?

(A) Positive and Negative Syndrome Scale (PANSS).

(B) Brief Psychiatric Rating Scale (BPRS).

(C) Scale for The Assessment of Positive Symptoms (SAPS).

(D) Scale for The Assessment of Negative Symptoms (SANS).

(104) In which of the following mood disorders does the rating scale require clinician ratings and data obtained from informants?

(A) Bipolar disorder, current manic episode.

(B) Bipolar disorder, current depressive episode.

(C) Bipolar disorder, in remission.

(D) Major depressive disorder.

(105) Which of the following scales is used to assess somatic complaints in depression?

(A) Beck Depression Inventory (BDI).

(B) Hamilton Rating Scale for Depression (HAM-D).

(C) Clinician-Administered PTSD Scale (CAPS).

(D) The Brief Psychiatric Rating Scale (BPRS).

(106) The Hamilton Rating Scale for Depression may be problematic to use in which circumstance?

(A) Patients who suffer from depression and a personality disorder.

(B) Patients who suffer from depression and an anxiety disorder.

(C) Patients who suffer from depression and a medical illness.

(D) Adolescents who suffer from depression.

(107) Which of the following scales can be used to diagnose PTDS?

(A) Yale-Brown Obsessive-Compulsive Scale (YBOCS).

(B) Clinician-Administered PTSD Scale (CAPS).

(C) Panic Disorder Severity Scale (PDSS).

(D) Hamilton Anxiety Rating Scale (HAM-A).

(108) Which of the following scales can measure OCD symptom severity?

(A) Yale-Brown Obsessive-Compulsive Scale (YBOCS).

(B) Clinician-Administered PTSD Scale (CAPS).

(C) Panic Disorder Severity Scale (PDSS).

(D) Hamilton Anxiety Rating Scale (HAM-A).

(109) Which of the following scales can be used as a screening instrument for depression?

(A) Beck Depression Inventory (BDI).

(B) Hamilton Rating Scale for Depression (HAM-D).

(C) Clinician-Administered PTSD Scale (CAPS).

(D) The Brief Psychiatric Rating Scale (BPRS).

(110) A 34-year-old patient who suffers from panic disorder reports that recently he has started enjoying alcohol. He says that during his young years he never had a drink. Which scale should you administer to assess for a potential alcohol problem?

(A) Mini-Mental State Examination (MMSE).

(B) Brief Psychiatric Rating Scale (BPRS).

(C) Addiction Severity Index (ASI).

(D) CAGE.

(111) A 42-year-old male patient with a five-year intravenous drug use history complains of depressed mood and lack of appetite. Which psychiatric rating scale should be administered to assess the functional impairment caused by the drug use?

(A) Hamilton Rating Scale for Depression (HAM-D).

(B) CAGE.

(C) Addiction Severity Index (ASI).

(D) Beck Depression Inventory (BDI).

(112) Which of the following can be a barrier to communication?

(A) The size of the room.

(B) The lighting in the room.

(C) Time constraints.

(D) The number of staff in the hospital.

(113) During a group therapy session, you are called because a suicidal patient you have been treating is experiencing major distress. What is the best course of action in this situation?

(A) Finish the group therapy session and then see the suicidal patient.

(B) Request that someone else see the patient.

(C) Leave the session without telling the group therapy patients why you left.

(D) Explain to the group therapy patients that you must leave and arrange the time when you will be coming back.

(114) During a session with a young female patient who is suffering from panic disorder, you notice that she is nodding while you are talking to her, but she does not seem to understand what you are saying. Outside the room, there is a lot of noise from the kindergarten next to the hospital. What could be the cause of the patient's difficulty in understanding?

(A) The patient's cognitive abilities.

(B) The patient's anxiety.

(C) The background noise.

(D) The patient's mental health literacy.

(115) Which of the following is not a way to overcome the effect of noise on communication?

(A) Yelling at the patient.

(B) Going to a quieter room.

(C) Finding a quiet corner.

(D) Checking if the patient's hearing aids are working properly.

(116) Which of the following patients may have trouble completing a written form?

(A) A 34-year-old female patient with bulimia nervosa who is in session with her mother.

(B) A 27-year-old male patient with schizophrenia who is not in a psychotic episode.

(C) A 23-year-old Latino patient with Generalized Anxiety Disorder (GAD) who does not understand English very well.

(D) A 15-year-old male patient with attention-deficit/hyperactivity disorder (ADHD).

(117) What is the most appropriate way to approach a patient who is in distress when you have to obtain information from them?

(A) Ask them directly about the information you need.

(B) Acknowledge their discomfort and express that it is important to talk.

(C) Wait until their discomfort is over.

(D) Give them a written form.

(118) How can you make the information easier to process when a patient is unable to give their full attention?

(A) By breaking down the information into smaller parts.

(B) By writing down the information.

(C) By talking to a friend or a family member, instead of the patient.

(D) By using an interpreter.

(119) Which of the following is an obvious sign of embarrassment?

(A) Joking.

(B) Fidgeting.

(C) Laughter.

(D) Blushing.

(120) Which of the following is an example of a non-judgmental question?

(A) You did not drink before you came to the interview, right?

(B) You do know that your drug use is affecting your academic success?

(C) When was the last time you had a glass of wine?

(D) You haven't used heroin in the past week, have you?

(121) Which of the following statements is false regarding the effect of embarrassment and anxiety on effective communication?

(A) Patients may feel embarrassed when having to talk about sensitive information like difficult family situations, addictions, sexual dysfunction, etc.

(B) You should avoid judgmental statements since they increase embarrassment.

(C) Patients have no issues asking for clarification when they have trouble understanding something.

(D) Signs of embarrassment include laughter, fidgeting, joking, and blushing.

(122) What is the purpose of using medical jargon and clinical acronyms?

(A) To make communication between healthcare providers and patients easier.

(B) To make communication between healthcare providers easier.

(C) To hide sensitive information from patients.

(D) To overcomplicate unnecessarily.

(123) When you are taking care of a patient who is not fluent in English, you can help them understand you better by doing what?

(A) Using complex sentences.

(B) Incorporating slang terms.

(C) Talking slowly.

(D) Presenting information with statistics.

(124) A male nurse practitioner is taking care of a patient who believes that nurse practitioners should be only female. What should the nurse practitioner do to overcome this barrier?

(A) Introduce himself and his role.

(B) Transfer the patient to another female nurse practitioner.

(C) Ignore the patient's assumptions.

(D) Stop taking care of the patient.

(125) Which of the following is not used to prevent information overload?

(A) Taking notes during the session.

(B) Recording the conversation.

(C) Providing patients with written information.

(D) Calling the patient at random times during the day if you remember additional information.

(126) What does paralanguage consist of?

(A) Speaking and writing.

(B) Facial expression, body posture, eye movements, and touch.

(C) Speed of speech, intonation, voice quality, and rhythm.

(D) Speaking, writing, facial expression, body posture, eye movements, and touch.

(127) Which of the following is not recommended when using an interpreter with a patient who is not fluent in English?

(A) Keeping eye contact with the patient.

(B) Speaking to the interpreter and not directly to the patient.

(C) Speaking directly to the patient instead of speaking to the interpreter.

(D) Discussing emotional and intimate topics.

(128) Which of the following statements is false regarding communication with the use of an interpreter?

(A) You should use technical jargon when talking to the interpreter.

(B) If there is a possibility, you can allow the patient and interpreter to meet before the interview to build rapport.

(C) Before starting emotional and intimate topics, you should ask the patient for permission.

(D) Before starting emotional and intimate topics, you should ask the interpreter for permission.

(129) When using an interpreter during a conversation with a patient who is not fluent in English what is best in terms of the interpreter?

(A) To be of the same gender and similar age as the patient.

(B) To be of the same culture as the patient.

(C) To be of the same religion as the patient.

(D) To share the same political beliefs as the patient.

(130) What is a common belief in collectivist cultures regarding personal failures?

(A) Failures are due to individual weaknesses.

(B) Failures are seen as learning opportunities.

(C) Failures occur because of external circumstances.

(D) Failures are inevitable and unchangeable.

(131) Which of the following statements is false regarding the influence of culture on communication?

(A) Some cultures consider silence as passive aggression.

(B) The patient's culture may influence the extent of their self-disclosure.

(C) Patients with different cultural backgrounds use the same terms to describe mental illness.

(D) Eye contact is considered disrespectful in some cultural groups.

(132) The Neuropsychiatric Inventory is an interview that is performed by a trained interviewer or a clinician with a caregiver or other informant. There is a version for a nursing home interview (NPI-NH) and a self-report questionnaire (NPI-Q). For every area, the NPI first asks if the symptom is present. The NPI is used in the assessment of what?

(A) Cognitive symptoms of major depressive disorder (MDD).

(B) Behavioral symptoms in dementia.

(C) Affective symptoms of obsessive-compulsive disorder (OCD).

(D) Emotional regulation in borderline personality disorder (BPD).

(133) Which of the following statements is correct regarding the psychiatric rating scales used in the assessment of cognitive disorders?

(A) The Mini-Mental State Examination (MMSE) is used in the assessment of behavioral symptoms in Alzheimer's disease and other types of dementia.

(B) The Mini-Mental State Examination (MMSE) is used in the assessment of somatic symptoms in Alzheimer's disease and other types of dementia.

(C) The Scored General Intelligence Test (SGIT) is used to measure affective symptoms of Alzheimer's disease and other types of dementia.

(D) The Mini-Mental State Examination (MMSE) is a cognitive test that that is used to assess cognitive functions in many domains (orientation, memory, language, attention, and construction).

(134) Quality and safety improvement initiatives are necessary in healthcare. Most medical errors occur due to which of the following?

(A) Imperfections of the medical education system.

(B) Negligence.

(C) Personality traits of healthcare providers.

(D) Imperfections of processes and systems.

(135) The quality of healthcare can be measured by assessing its structure, processes, and outcomes. The structure of healthcare determines the accessibility and availability of resources, as well as their quality. The structure of healthcare includes which of the following?

(A) The number of nurses with appropriate education and training, the number of beds in the hospital, and health insurance.

(B) The delivery of healthcare services by healthcare providers.

(C) The usage of up-to-date guidelines.

(D) Patient satisfaction, health status, morbidity, and mortality.

(136) What is the approach that aims to improve quality based on the premise that, to achieve the best outcome, the whole organization should commit to quality?

(A) Frequent Quality Improvement.

(B) Continuous Quality Improvement.

(C) Regular Quality Improvement.

(D) Punctual Quality Improvement.

(137) Which of the following is not a part of the quality improvement process?

(A) Identifying a process that needs to be improved.

(B) Measuring factors involved in key programs.

(C) Incorporation of beliefs and values in the improvement process.

(D) Reassessments to determine whether the change has resulted in an improved process.

(138) Providing reminder systems can be achieved by what?

(A) Giving performance feedback to individual providers.

(B) Publicly releasing performance data.

(C) Incorporating reminders in charts for providers.

(D) Distributing educational material and content.

(139) Which of the following quality improvement models is used for rapid cycle improvement?

(A) Six Sigma.

(B) The Plan-Do-Study-Act (PDSA)

(C) Root-cause analysis.

(D) Lean.

(140) Which of the following statements is false regarding adverse events in healthcare?

(A) Medical errors and failures in patient safety are an issue of healthcare quality that can be responsible for patient death.

(B) The complexity and imperfection of the healthcare delivery system are responsible for most medical lapses.

(C) Adverse events are overreported.

(D) Adverse events rarely occur because of negligence or medical malpractice.

(141) Which of the following statements is false regarding the list of serious reportable adverse events?

(A) The main purpose of the list of serious reportable events is to identify a standard set of adverse events that would increase public accountability for their occurrence.

(B) When an adverse event occurs, oversight bodies should investigate the causes behind it.

(C) Healthcare providers do not have public accountability to provide information about their performance and actions to the public.

(D) Oversight bodies exist to make sure that providers are compliant with accepted standards of care.

(142) Which of the following is not part of the criteria of the list of serious reportable adverse events?

(A) It should be clearly measurable and identifiable.

(B) It should be significantly influenced by the clinician's education.

(C) It should be preventable, the majority of the time.

(D) It should pose a concern to the public and healthcare providers.

(143) Which of the following statements is false regarding the list of serious reportable adverse events?

(A) The list of adverse events includes criminal events.

(B) Healthcare facilities should eliminate all risk of adverse events.

(C) The list of serious reportable adverse events is organized in six categories.

(D) The list of serious reportable adverse events is short due to the belief that a clearly defined, short list will be more easily understood.

(144) Which of the following does not influence patient's expectations of the treatment outcome?

(A) The patient's personality.

(B) Previous experiences with mental health treatment.

(C) The clinician's ethnic background.

(D) Information the patient has obtained through the media or others.

(145) The clinician should consider the physical and psychological symptoms of the disorder that may interfere with the treatment they plan to prescribe. A patient who has suffered a stroke and is limited in their mobility because of paralysis may have difficulties with what?

(A) Therapeutic techniques that involve verbal expression.

(B) Therapeutic techniques that involve introspection.

(C) Therapeutic behavioral techniques.

(D) Therapeutic cognitive techniques.

(146) Which therapeutic technique involves verbal expression to help patients process their thoughts and emotions?

(A) Cognitive Behavioral Therapy.

(B) Art Therapy.

(C) Music Therapy.

(D) Dance/Movement Therapy.

(147) The number of referrals from nonpsychiatric medical professions has increased because of which reason?

(A) Patients are unsatisfied with the care they receive from nonpsychiatric medical professionals.

(B) It is mandatory to refer patients to psychiatry.

(C) Patients ask to see a psychiatrist.

(D) Healthcare providers have become more sensitive to psychiatric issues in their patients.

(148) Systematically developed declarations that support certain treatment actions or approaches are called what?

(A) Treatment manuals.

(B) Clinical practice guidelines.

(C) Empirically supported treatments.

(D) Educational materials.

(149) Which of the following is a disadvantage of treatment manuals?

(A) They increase face-to-face interaction between providers and patients.

(B) They provide an opportunity for education.

(C) They tend to involve mechanical implementation which makes them inflexible and nonintuitive.

(D) They demonstrate effectiveness and achievement of positive outcomes in randomized controlled trials.

(150) The integration of the best available research combined with clinical experience is called what?

(A) Treatment manuals.

(B) Randomized Controlled Trials.

(C) Clinical Practice Guidelines.

(D) Empirically Supported Treatments.

Test 3: Answers and Explanations

(1) (D) Develop positive mental health for individuals with mental health problems and the community in general.

Promotion of mental health can help people manage life situations and events more easily, whether they are predictable or unpredictable. Mental health promotion can help patients increase their self-esteem and well-being. Health promotion involves working with individuals, groups, and communities. The psychiatric mental-health nurse practitioner teaches people to improve life skills as well as their quality of life.

(2) (A) Reducing hospital readmissions.

The main goal of disease management is to reduce hospital readmissions by providing comprehensive and continuous care that helps patients manage their conditions effectively.

(3) (C) People that are without, at risk of, or with mental illness.

Mental health promotion is focused on advocating for the emotional and social well-being of people without mental illness, people who are at risk of mental illness, and people who experience mental illness. Goals of health promotion include protection, support, and sustainability of social and emotional well-being, promotion of mentally healthy lifestyles, and support of productive and meaningful lives. Mental health promotion aims to increase people's sense of belonging and connectedness.

(4) (A) Relapse prevention.

Relapse prevention is not one of the goals of mental health prevention. The goals of mental health promotion include building resilience by increasing protective factors and reducing risk factors that can be threatening to emotional and social well-being, increasing people's sense of belonging and connectedness, improving coping skills and adaptations of individuals and communities, especially in the face of adversity, enabling healthy communities, workplaces, schools, and social supports and building community acceptance and tolerance by increasing the understanding of cultural, personal, social, and spiritual differences.

(5) (B) Mental health prevention.

Mental health prevention can be defined as interventions that are done before the onset of a mental illness that aim to prevent its development. These interventions can target specific life stages to reduce the development of mental illness during lifecycle transitions and age-associated onset. Prevention can target the individual or populations. It can be divided into primary, secondary, and tertiary prevention.

(6) (D) Minimize the incidence and prevalence of certain psychiatric disorders.

The main goals of mental health prevention are to reduce the incidence and prevalence of certain psychiatric disorders (primary and secondary prevention), to reduce or delay the recurrence, frequency, and interval of psychiatric disorders (relapse prevention), and to reduce the time a patient spends with a psychiatric disorder, reduce the impact and severity of the disorder, and the distress, pain, and suffering associated with the psychiatric disorder (treatment, recovery, secondary, and tertiary prevention).

(7) (A) Prevent or reduce the recurrence of a disorder and the exacerbation of symptoms.

Relapse prevention helps people stay in a good state after a first or subsequent episode of a psychiatric disorder. Relapse prevention aims to prevent or reduce the recurrence of a disorder, and symptom exacerbation. Relapse prevention includes medication adherence and psychoeducation, as well as promotion of awareness, resilience, and recovery. What happens to the patient while they are in remission can have a big impact on prevention.

(8) (B) Policy changes, social action, and economic management.

Policy changes, social action, and economic management are a part of mental health promotion on a community level, while relapse prevention is done on an individual level. The successful relapse prevention plan consists of increased awareness, behavioral change, identification of the relapse signature, mutual collaboration between the healthcare staff, identification of the patient's personal preference, maintenance, early intervention, empowerment, and resilience.

(9) (C) Resilience depends only on the patient's constitution.

Resilience is an interactive dynamic process that emerges as a product of the environment the person is living in and their constitution. Patients differ in their ability to cope with adverse situations and avoid breaking down when confronted with stressful events. Responses to stress are often coping mechanisms. Coping and defensive mechanisms can be healthy or maladaptive.

(10) (C) Early in the mental health assessment process.

Identifying risk factors for mental illness is an important component in the development of resilience. Risk factors should be identified early in the psychosocial and mental health assessment. They can help the clinician determine risk management, scope of intervention, and care planning. Identification of risk factors can help strengthen resilience at both the individual and community level.

(11) (C) A positive temperament.

A positive temperament is a protective factor against mental illness, not a risk factor. Common risk factors include poor or interrupted development or maturity, unstable and dysfunctional interpersonal relationships, absent or poor parenting, family discord, domestic violence and abuse, parent(s) with severe psychiatric disorder and disability, overwhelming adversity or grief and loss, loneliness, lack of peer and social support, lack of friends, drug or alcohol use, poor nutrition, poor sleep, social exclusion, social disadvantage, injustice, poverty, stigma, and persistent physical disability.

(12) (A) Anti-bullying programs in schools.

At the community level, resilience and protective factors can be promoted through anti-bullying programs in schools, healthy working environments, promotion of healthy lifestyles, self-help, and personal growth, development courses, mental health literacy, teaching people about emotional intelligence, and connecting people in the community with ethnic minorities and the socially disadvantaged. Building resilience at the community level increases emotional well-being in society.

(13) (C) Poor nutrition.

Poor nutrition is a risk factor for mental illness. Common protective factors include a healthy lifestyle, nurturing and affectionate family relationships, positive school and work environments, social "connectedness" and belonging, reliable friendships and social support networks, a positive "temperament" (humor, patience, hope, and tolerance), emotional intelligence, self-awareness, self-esteem, acceptance, opportunities and achievements, and the presence of mentors or personal encouragements.

(14) (D) Buproprion.

Nicotine is among the most addictive substances and can be very difficult to quit. Tobacco cessation may require multiple attempts and different methods. Varenicline and bupropion are non-nicotine-based medications that can be helpful for long-term cessation. There are nicotine-based medications that are used as nicotine-replacement therapy. A combination of counseling and medication is more effective than either alone.

(15) (C) Provide them with nicotine-replacement therapy.

Tobacco use should be assessed in patients who are admitted to the hospital. During hospitalization, patients who are addicted to nicotine will experience withdrawal symptoms if they do not have access to nicotine-replacement products. Therefore, they should be provided nicotine-replacement therapy, such as nicotine gums or patches.

(16) (B) Every patient who is admitted.

Assessment of tobacco use should be done for every patient at admission. Nurses should ask every smoker whether they have an intention to quit smoking. If they do, refer them to services that help with cessation. Encourage the use of apps and quit lines and offer health education to every tobacco user. Every patient should have an individualized quitting plan.

(17) (C) Problem-focused coping.

Problem-focused coping is most effective for managing extreme stress as it involves actively addressing the source of stress through strategies such as seeking information, planning, and taking direct action.

(18) (C) At least 30 minutes every day.

You should advise patients to get regular exercise for at least 30 minutes per day. Regular exercise is known to improve mood, mental health, and cognitive abilities.

Patients should also be advised to eat healthy and balanced meals with regular hydration. This will improve their focus and increase their energy throughout the day. They should also limit caffeinated beverages and beverages with high sugar content.

(19) (D) Watch TV shows before bed.

Patients should be educated about the importance of sleep. Watching TV shows before bed is not beneficial for sleep and can negatively impact it.

(20) (C) A person who has been eating poorly for the past month and has unexpectedly lost six pounds.

Inform patients that they should seek professional help if they have experienced severe symptoms for two weeks or more. Distressing and severe symptoms include difficulty sleeping, changes in appetite that have resulted in weight gain or loss, struggle to get out of bed due to mood changes, issues with concentration and focus, issues with daily functioning, and a loss of interest in previously enjoyable activities.

(21) (D) A 34-year-old male patient who comes to the hospital for the first time because he is having trouble falling asleep for the past month.

A sleep disorder is not an emergency psychiatric situation. Psychiatric emergencies require immediate therapeutic intervention. Emergency psychiatry deals with issues such as violence (homicide, suicide, and rape), substance abuse, abuse of children and spouses, and social issues (competence, homelessness, and aging). The most common diagnoses seen in the psychiatric emergency department are mood disorders (depression and manic episodes), schizophrenia, and alcohol dependence.

(22) (C) Medical conditions do not present with emergency psychiatric manifestations.

One-third of medical conditions may present with psychiatric manifestations. Therefore, the staff should have access to the medical emergency department.

(23) (B) A 34-year-old male patient with major depressive disorder reports that he is planning to kill himself because life is not worth living.

Certain modifications in the standard psychiatric evaluation when dealing with an emergency psychiatry situation may be necessary. When assessing a patient's risk of suicide, the usual rules of confidentiality may need to be abandoned, especially if the patient is a danger to themselves.

(24) (D) Talk to him in a calm voice and say, "You will not harm anyone."

If there is a risk of violence, the patient should first be reassured and calmed in a non-threatening way. Use any methods that may be necessary to prevent the patient from injuring themselves, including physical restraint. Violence towards others must also be prevented. First, the patient's risk of violence should be assessed. Medication should be offered if verbal de-escalation fails. When both pharmacotherapy and verbal de-escalation fail, the staff may be required to use physical restraints.

(25) (D) Young age at onset.

Factors that point towards a medical cause of a psychiatric presentation include acute onset, older age at onset, the first episode, the presence of a comorbid medical illness or injury, nonauditory hallucinations, mental status signs (e.g., disorientation, reduced alertness, impairment of memory, concentration, and attention, speech problems), history of significant substance abuse, neurologic symptoms (e.g., loss of consciousness, change in vision, head injury, seizures), and constructional apraxia (e.g., the patient is struggling to draw a clock).

(26) (B) Diabetic ketoacidosis.

Emergency situations can have medical, psychiatric, or both medical and psychiatric etiology. Medical conditions that cause mental status changes that resemble mental illness include diabetes mellitus, acute intoxications, withdrawal, thyroid disease, AIDS, and head traumas. Medical conditions can be life-threatening and they generally have a more definitive treatment with a better prognosis.

(27) (A) Antisocial Personality Disorder.

The differential diagnosis of violent behavior is wide and it includes medical causes (cerebral neoplasms, infections, temporal robe epilepsy), personality disorders (antisocial personality disorders, paranoid personality disorder, decompensating obsessive-compulsive personality disorder), dissociative disorders, delusional disorder, bipolar disorder, violence due to interpersonal stress, schizophrenia, psychoactive substance-induced organic mental disorder, alcohol intoxication, and others.

(28) (A) Psychomotor retardation.

Certain signs that might alert the clinician of impending violence include recent acts of violence, history of violent behavior, threats (verbal or physical), progressive psychomotor agitation, alcohol or drug intoxication, persecutory ideation in a psychotic patient, catatonic excitement, history of violent acts, and a history of childhood abuse.

(29) (C) A homeless 28-year-old male patient with a substance abuse problem.

The demographic is an important factor when assessing the risk for violence since violent patients are most often young male patients with a low socioeconomic status and few social supports. Other factors that should be considered include violent ideation. Patients with a history of violence, nonviolent antisocial acts, and low impulse control have an increased risk of violence. The presence of interpersonal stressor in the patient's life (e.g., marital conflict) is another important predictor.

(30) (A) Agitation.

Agitation is usually associated with an underlying medical or psychiatric condition. Violence can result from aggression or agitation. Aggression is less likely to be due to a mental disorder. The psychiatric interview can be used as a screening tool to determine whether threats of violence have a psychiatric origin.

(31) (D) Verbal de-escalation.

De-escalation is the primary goal in dealing with an agitated patient. Verbal de-escalation is attempted at first. Simple sentences are helpful since they are more likely to be understood by confused patients. Pharmacologic medication with benzodiazepines or antipsychotics can be used if verbal de-escalation fails. If both measures fail, the staff may be required to use physical restraints. Restraints should be used only in extreme circumstances since they cause both physical and psychological trauma.

(32) (D) Every patient should be asked if they have thoughts of suicide.

All psychiatric disorders increase the risk of suicide. During the mental state examination, the clinician should directly ask every patient who presents with a mental health concern if they have suicidal thoughts or ideas. The majority of patients with intent to commit suicide give warning about their plan. Therefore, direct questions (e.g., Are you suicidal?) should be regularly asked to assess suicidality risk.

(33) (C) The presence of an anxiety disorder.

Signs that indicate an increased risk of suicide include a history of suicidal attempt(s), a history of suicidal ideation, availability of means of suicide, a family history, pervasive pessimism or hopelessness, a concern for the effect of suicide on family members, verbalized suicidal ideation, life crisis, preparation of a will, admitting to a plan of action, and resignation after agitated depression (e.g., a patient who was previously threatening suicide suddenly becomes quiet).

(34) (A) Hospitalize the patient and have him monitored 24/7.

This patient has an increased risk of suicide (admits to a plan, concerned for the effect of suicide on family members). Patients who have an imminent risk of suicidal behavior must be hospitalized or protected in another way. Involuntary hospitalization may be needed in patients who are a danger to themselves. Hospitalized patients may need intensive monitoring and observation which may include the presence of a one-to-one "sitter."

(35) (D) The nurse should not perform a physical examination on a patient who presents with suicidal ideation since that might make them extremely uncomfortable.

A physical examination should be done on all patients who present with suicidal ideation to search for signs of self-injurious behavior (e.g., if the patient has cut themselves). In the inpatient setting, you must make sure that the patient does not have access to any means by which they can harm themselves such as glass or other sharp items.

(36) (A) Toxicology screen.

A toxicology screen should be done on this patient to assess for occult overdose. Patients who come to the hospital with suicidal ideation may have already attempted it by ingesting substances to overdose. Since the effects of overdose are not apparent in the first hours after ingestion, you should order labs (e.g., acetylsalicylic acid level) to assess for an occult overdose.

(37) (D) Grandiose delusions.

Factors that increase the likelihood of a suicide attempt in the near future include access to guns, use of ethanol or other substances that increase impulsivity, recent suicide attempt(s), ongoing thoughts of suicide, and recent self-harm.

(38) (C) Rape victims are never male.

Though the majority of victims are female, male rape also occurs. Normal reactions in victims include humiliation, shame, anxiety, confusion, and outrage. Many victims feel partially responsible for the assault. The clinician who is evaluating a rape and sexual abuse victim should provide reassurance and support in a nonjudgmental way.

(39) (C) Diazepam.

Intoxication from drugs of abuse can be treated with conservative measures. Haloperidol is given 5 to 10 mg every half-hour to an hour in certain patients who need to be stabilized. If the drug that caused the intoxication has anticholinergic properties, it is better to use benzodiazepines instead of antipsychotics.

(40) (A) 5 to 10 mg Diazepam slowly and intravenously.

For violent patients, you may give 5 to 10 mg Diazepam or 2 to 4 mg Lorazepam, slowly and intravenously over two minutes. In administration of IV medication, the nurse should take great care to avoid causing respiratory arrest.

(41) (B) Regular clinical assessments.

Regular clinical assessments are the best method to evaluate the effectiveness of treatment because they provide objective, consistent, and comprehensive data on the patient's progress and response to treatment.

(42) (B) A stagnation of the patient's condition.

Choosing the inappropriate level of care can cause stagnation or worsening of the patient's condition. Specific tools that help clinicians decide the appropriate LOC can be used. For example, the Aetna's Level of Care Assessment Tool (LOCAT) helps healthcare providers determine the LOC for patients with psychiatric disorders.

(43) (A) Conjoined marital therapy.

Psychotherapeutic formats include individual therapy, group therapy, family therapy, etc. Some patients benefit the most from individual therapy. Some patients may see the best results from group therapy. The optimal type of psychotherapy depends on a number of factors. For example, a patient who is seeking help for their marital problems will most likely benefit the most from conjoint marital therapy.

(44) (B) Group therapy.

A patient who has problems connecting and relating to others will benefit most from group therapy. For some patients, the best approach would be a combination of modalities (e.g., individual and family therapy), while for others the preferred approach is a succession of modalities (e.g., sessions of individual psychotherapy followed by ten sessions of family therapy).

(45) (C) A patient with marital problems.

A patient who is seeking help for their marital problems will most likely benefit from conjoined marital therapy. Many patients present with symptoms that cannot be alleviated without psychopharmacologic interventions. Psychopharmacologic intervention is a good approach for patients who suffer from major depressive disorder, attention-deficit/hyperactivity disorder, or psychotic disorders.

(46) (A) A patient with major depressive disorder.

Many patients present with symptoms that cannot be alleviated without psychopharmacologic interventions. Medications are the most effective treatments for some disorders, either alone or in combination with another therapeutic modality. Psychopharmacologic intervention is a good approach for patients who suffer from major depressive disorder, attention-deficit/hyperactivity disorder, or psychotic disorders.

(47) (A) A patient with major depressive disorder.

Many patients present with symptoms that cannot be alleviated without psychopharmacologic interventions. Medications are the most effective treatments for some disorders, either alone or in combination with another therapeutic modality. Psychopharmacologic intervention is a good approach for patients who suffer from major depressive disorder, attention-deficit/hyperactivity disorder, or psychotic disorders.

(48) (B) Treatments with a wide focus are more effective than highly focused treatments.

Most psychotherapy treatments are effective, However, some are more effective than others. For example, highly focused treatments (e.g., systemic desensitization for the treatment of phobias) are more effective than treatments with a wide focus (e.g., client-centered care in the development of personal growth goals). Factors that influence treatment effectiveness include the specific therapy techniques, the patient's expectations of the outcome, the patient's characteristics, the patient's circumstances and environment, and others.

(49) (C) Ethnic background.

The clinical expertise of the clinician who is treating the patient consists of his/her diagnostic competence, clinical decision-making, case formulation, treatment planning and implementation, monitoring of progress, interpersonal skills, incorporation of new knowledge and skills, and continuous self-reflection. A clinician with a high clinical expertise has a higher chance of achieving a good outcome.

(50) (A) Cultural consideration.

The patient's culture needs to be taken into consideration when prescribing and beginning treatment. Certain guidelines can help clinicians practice cultural adaptation in the treatment process. The services that clinicians provide should be meaningful in the cultural context in which they are being delivered. Before implementing treatment, clinicians should conduct cultural assessments. They should use traditional treatments as existing resources and communicate in a culturally appropriate empathetic manner.

(51) (B) Role preferences.

The majority of patients want to actively participate in the treatment plan development and make decisions. Clinicians should be aware of patients' preferences. Role preferences refer to the expectations that patients have from the clinician's behavior. Some patients prefer that the therapist provides a listening role whereas others prefer a more active advice-giving role.

(52) (C) Therapist preferences.

Clinicians should be aware of patients' preferences. Therapist preferences refer to those related to the clinician's characteristics. For example, some patients prefer that the therapist comes from a similar ethnic background. Some patients prefer therapists who have many years of clinical experience whereas others prefer younger therapists.

(53) (A) Treatment preferences.

Patients can have three types of preferences: role, therapist, and treatment-type preferences. Treatment preferences refer to those related to the specific type of intervention that the patient is expecting to receive. Some patients prefer a behavioral approach whereas others prefer a cognitive approach. Some prefer a pharmacological approach whereas some expect the best results from a psychotherapeutic approach. Patient preferences have a major role in the treatment outcome.

(54) (B) Negligence.

Medical malpractice is a civil wrong that results from negligence. Negligence means that the clinician who has a duty to care for patients has failed to do something they should or done something they should not as defined by the current medical practice.

(55) (D) The patient was damaged because of a deviation from the standard of care.

In order to prove malpractice, the plaintiff (e.g., the patient or their family) should obtain evidence that there was a (1) doctor-patient relationship and the doctor had a duty to care for the patient (duty), (2) there was a deviation from the standard of care (deviation), (3) the patient was injured or damaged (damage), (4) the deviation from the standard of care is what directly caused the damage (direct causation).

(56) (D) When the psychiatrist prescribes a medication that is not indicated for the patient's disorder, the patient's condition worsens as a consequence.

In order to find liability, each element of a malpractice claim should be present. For example, a psychiatrist cannot be liable for malpractice if there is no doctor-patient relationship that created duty of care, even if the psychiatrist's negligence causes direct harm to a patient. Psychiatrists are not liable if they give advice on social media or television programs since there is no doctor-patient relationship in general advice-giving.

(57) (B) A bad outcome of the patient's condition.

Psychiatrists are not liable for malpractice if the patient's worsening condition is not related to negligence. Every bad outcome is not caused by negligence. Other than negligence, patients can sue for false imprisonment, intentional tort of assault, defamation, battery, fraud, intentional infliction of emotional distress, and misrepresentation. Intentional tort means that the psychiatrist has done something that they realize, or should have realized, would bring harm to the patient.

(58) (C) When a clinician uses a drug-interaction checker before prescribing medication.

Negligent prescription practice occurs when a clinician exceeds the recommended doses, does not adjust the medication levels to therapeutic, prescribes not-indicated medications, mixes medications unreasonably, does not disclose medication effects and prescribes too many medications at the same time. Older patients take many medications prescribed by various physicians. When prescribing psychotropic medications, special care should be taken to avoid harmful interactions and side effects. The prescribing clinician should document their reasons for prescribing multiple medications.

(59) (A) The prescribing clinician has no responsibility to give detailed information about the medications they are prescribing.

There is no consistently accepted standard for what information should be disclosed in a psychiatric or medical situation. Generally, the clinician should provide the patient with a description of their condition, the nature and goal of the proposed treatment, the risks and benefits of the treatment, possible alternatives to the treatment, their risks and benefits, and prognosis about the outcome with and without treatment.

(60) (D) After every medication change.

Informed consent should be obtained after every medication change or after introducing a new drug. Obtaining informed consent from a patient can be difficult if the patient has a reduced cognitive capacity due to mental illness or neurological disease. A substitute caretaker can provide consent in these situations. If the doctor does not inform the patient of the risks associated with the medication and the medication injures the patient, there is sufficient ground for a malpractice claim.

(61) (B) To ensure medication compliance and monitor side effects.

A follow-up interval of one month is usually recommended to ensure that patients are compliant with their medication regimen and to monitor for any potential side effects or adverse reactions.

(62) (C) Split treatment.

Split treatment occurs when a psychiatrist prescribes medication and another nonmedical therapist provides psychotherapy. Split treatment causes fragmented care and may have dangerous consequences. The psychiatrist has the responsibility to be fully informed of the patient's status at all times. The psychiatrist should be informed of the quality and type of therapy the nonmedical therapist provides. When the relationship between the psychiatrist and nonmedical therapist is collaborative, they both take responsibility for the patient's care.

(63) (B) Providing continuous monitoring for safety.

When a patient is placed in seclusion, continuous monitoring is essential to ensure their safety and to observe any changes in their condition. This helps to prevent harm to the patient and ensures that their physical and emotional needs are being met during the period of seclusion.

(64) (C) If the patient's condition poses a risk to themselves or others.

A patient's visitation rights can be restricted if their condition poses a risk to themselves or others. In such cases, the clinician must document the reasons for restricting visitation.

(65) (A) A patient who has criminal charges of threatening phone calls.

Open and free communication with the world outside is allowed, by phone or mail, but there may be exceptions. In certain cases, jurisdictions charge hospitals with the duty to monitor the patients' communications. Patients with criminal charges of threatening or harassing phone calls should not be allowed unrestricted access to the phone. Patients are allowed to have private telephone calls, and the staff should not invade their privacy by listening to their conversations.

(66) (D) A 67-year-old delirious patient with dementia.

Seclusion and restraint have specific indications and contraindications. A patient can be secluded or restrained if they pose harm to themselves or others. Patients who are extremely unstable, delirious, demented, or overtly suicidal should not be secluded except if they are closely monitored and supervised. The condition of a secluded and restrained patient must be regularly observed, documented, and reviewed. Their vital signs, nutrition, elimination, and hydration should be assessed every ten to fifteen minutes.

(67) (D) When a mentally incompetent patient is in an emergency situation.

In certain situations, the patient's refusal of treatment can be dismissed. Examples include when the patient is mentally incompetent to decide and the treatment is required to save their life or avoid severe harm, or if the refusal of treatment puts another's life or health in danger. In emergency situations, if the patient is not in a position to exercise judgment, the doctor does not have to obtain informed consent.

(68) (A) Their legal guardian.

If a patient is legally determined mentally incompetent, their legal guardian is the one who provides consent. In certain scenarios, a patient who is in a mental state that does not allow for informed decision-making (e.g., psychosis, unconsciousness) may not have a legal guardian. In these cases, consent should be obtained from the nearest relative. If the patient does not have a relative nearby, the clinician can ask the court to appoint a guardian.

(69) (B) Information about the treatment might cause a placebo effect.

Informed consent means that the patient has agreed to a specific treatment procedure after the healthcare provider has given enough information about the procedure, its risks, benefits, expected outcomes, and possible alternatives. In the case of a therapeutic privilege, the clinician withholds information because full disclosure may complicate or obstruct treatment, be too upsetting for the patient, or cause severe psychological harm.

(70) (B) If the patient needs immediate psychiatric treatment.

Temporary hospitalization can occur when a patient is acutely disturbed and is in need of immediate psychiatric treatment. This type of hospitalization requires a written recommendation from one clinician and confirmation from another psychiatrist or hospital staff.

(71) (A) A schizophrenic patient who is aware that he is hearing voices.

A person who is involuntarily hospitalized has significant restrictions on their rights and freedoms. Involuntary hospitalization may be required when the patient is a serious danger to themselves (suicidal) or others (homicidal), the patient is need for observation or treatment, or if the patient is unable to take care of their basic personal needs. The individual who is seeking involuntary hospitalization must have sufficient evidence to show why the patient is being hospitalized against their will.

(72) (C) The patient will be released.

Patients who are involuntarily hospitalized have the right to legal counsel. Their case can be brought before a judge. If the judge believes the patient should not be hospitalized, the patient is released. During the patient's stay, their case is reviewed periodically by a board that includes psychiatrists, lawyers, other physicians, and other citizens.

(73) (A) Written information that damages a person's reputation.

If shared information damages the patient's reputation, the person who shared the information can be liable for defamation of character. If the shared information is in written form, the liability is called libel. When the information is shared orally, it is called slander. Libel may occur when the patient's medical record contains critical or judgmental statements. Psychiatric nurses should back up everything they write in the chart with factual evidence.

(74) (B) Science.

The science component refers to the framework and support of the group which includes activities for planning, organizing, structuring, directing, and evaluating. The instructional part is necessary to achieve optimal functioning and group facilitation. The group leader should be skilled in basic interviewing, communication, and counseling. Skills are not a replacement for knowledge, understanding, and self-development of the group leader.

(75) (D) Techniques.

Techniques are strategies that help in teaching and group facilitation. Some techniques include activities like games, role-play, and exercises or teaching approaches such as discussions and media. Other examples of techniques are facilitating procedures like conflict resolution. Techniques can promote retention, participant involvement, and learning. Techniques should be used thoughtfully, and not as a replacement for reflection or a deeper understanding of personal issues and relationships.

(76) (A) It can prevent burnout and countertransference.

Personal development has a direct and indirect impact on clients. It can prevent burnout and countertransference, lead to a better understanding of client issues, and promote confidence about dealing with issues.

(77) (B) Transference.

Transference and countertransference are defined as processes through which one's individual thoughts, feelings, and wishes are transferred onto another person. Transference occurs when the process is transferred from a group member to the group leader. Countertransference occurs when the process is transferred from the group leader to the group member. These processes are unconscious and therefore can be hard to identify.

(78) (B) Countertransference.

Countertransference is a process that occurs when individual thoughts, feelings, and wishes are transferred from the group leader to the group member. Countertransference can be detrimental to the relationship with group members. It impacts the group leader's perception of the client, their reaction, the direction of sessions, and objectivity. Preventing countertransference can be achieved by bringing unresolved unconscious issues to conscious awareness and processing them.

(79) (C) Avoiding situations that cause anxiety.

Avoidant behavior involves deliberately avoiding situations or activities that cause anxiety or stress. This behavior can significantly impact daily functioning and quality of life.

(80) (D) Extreme professionalism without a sense of humor.

The group leader should have a sense of humor since laughing can relieve tension and promote a sense of playfulness. The group leader should have a deep belief in the group process. This will unconsciously provide reassurance and relief to the group members.

The group leader should have confidence in their group leadership abilities. They should be able to take risks and expose themselves to potential failures.

(81) (D) By learning about the group process and group dynamics.

Group leaders should understand the group as a whole and be able to respond timely as the session unfolds. Missing key events during sessions can have a negative impact on the group and make group members feel ignored. This can be prevented by learning about group dynamics, group stages, and helpful group factors. These components do not occur in isolation and they can change from moment to moment.

(82) (C) Group dynamics.

Group dynamics is the process of the group that includes the level of participation, resistance, relationship between members and between members and the leader, communication patterns, nonverbal behaviors, feelings expressed, and nonverbal behaviors.

(83) (A) The cooperation and interaction between members and the leader.

The cooperation and interaction between members and the leader, the contribution of members, and their functioning determines the level of participation. The group leader should observe the group dynamics since they can help determine the needs of the group members.

(84) (A) Over-participating member.

Members who over-participate will often interrupt other members while they are speaking. They may engage in distracting behaviors and monopolize the attention of the group leader. At the start of the process, it may be useful to have a member who over participates since they may engage and energize the other group members. However, their over-involvement usually becomes a problem. The group leader should find a way to reduce over participating behavior without offending the over participating member.

(85) (B) Socializing members.

Instead of participating in activities, socializers tend to start conversations and they are frequently late when coming back from breaks. One group usually has two or more socializers. In counseling/therapy groups, often the other group members may confront the socializers. You can deal with socializers by physically being near them, talking to them about their behavior, or making sure they are placed in different groups.

(86) (A) Under-participating members.

Under-participating members usually do the minimum required when participating in activities. Under-participating occurs as a self-protection or rebellion response. These members often did not choose to be in the group (e.g., court-ordered participants) and therefore, they refuse to participate in it. The group leader should not force them and should acknowledge that all members cannot be forced to participate. You can offer them opportunities that will give them the chance to involve themselves in the group but you cannot push them.

(87) (C) Disengaged member.

Disengaged members can disengage themselves from the group physically, mentally, or emotionally. Examples of physical disengagement include absence, being late, leaning back into the chair, or premature termination. An example of mental disengagement is daydreaming. Examples of emotional disengagement include changing the topic, not maintaining eye contact, asking rhetorical questions, intellectualizing, or becoming numb. Due to the short-term nature of psychoeducational groups, it may be hard to effectively manage disengaging behaviors.

(88) (D) Asking members to talk to each other directly.

You can encourage communication between members by asking them to talk to each other directly. Some members may be excluded from the communication. You can include them by asking for their input. Group members can communicate in a warm, supportive way or in a cold and hostile way. Some members appear aloof or tentative when they communicate. You should observe individual communication patterns as well as group patterns.

(89) (A) The group's overall emotional atmosphere.

The "feeling tone" of a therapeutic group refers to the overall emotional atmosphere within the group, which includes the collective emotions, moods, and attitudes of the group members. This tone can significantly influence the group's dynamics and the therapeutic process.

(90) (A) To provide individualized attention during group sessions.

Getting to know the group members individually allows you to tailor the therapeutic interventions to each member's unique needs, concerns, and personalities.

(91) (C) Start a discussion about the usefulness of the activity.

Resistance is a normal occurrence during the group process. When a group member shows resistance, you should move on to another topic or person. If the whole group is resistant, you can explore that by starting a discussion about the usefulness of the activity. You should not try to break down the resistance.

(92) (C) Psychiatric rating scales exist only in the format of questionnaires.

Psychiatric rating scales include questionnaires, checklists, outcome assessments, and other instruments that are used to inform psychiatric practice, research, and administration. Mental health providers should use psychiatric rating scales for several reasons. Psychiatric rating scales can be used to monitor the patient's progress over time. They can provide more information than a routine clinical interview.

(93) (B) Standardize information about the patient which has been collected by various providers.

The main goal of psychiatric rating scales is to standardize information about the patient which has been collected by various providers. By standardizing information, healthcare providers can have a comprehensive evaluation which can be used as an aid in treatment planning.

(94) (C) Predict whether the patient will experience any side effects in response to medication.

Psychiatric rating scales can help clinicians establish an accurate diagnosis, thoroughly describe symptoms, identify any potential comorbid conditions, and assess factors that impact treatment response. A rating scale can establish a baseline that will be used to monitor the progression of a disorder over time or in response to therapeutic interventions. This can be especially useful when more providers are caring for the patient such as in a group practice.

(95) (D) Constructs.

The broad ranges of areas that scales assess are referred to as constructs. Constructs can be diagnoses, quality of life, functional impairment, severity, signs, symptoms, etc. Some constructs are complex and need to be divided into a few domains such as positive and negative symptoms of schizophrenia. Constructs can be categorical (or classifying), continuous, or measuring.

(96) (A) Categorical.

Categorical constructs are used to describe whether a feature is currently present or absent (e.g., the ability to work a full-time job) or the category to which the patient belongs among other options (e.g., establishing a diagnosis).

(97) (B) Continuous.

Continuous scales are used to provide a quantitative assessment (measurement) of severity, frequency, or intensity. Continuous scales can measure cognitive status, multidimensional personality traits, symptom severity, functional status, and others.

(98) (A) The exact wordings of the questions that are asked are specified.

Scales are available in many formats that include checklists, self-administered questionnaires, tests, guides to observation, etc. Some scales are fully structured formal interviews. In a fully structured formal interview, the exact wordings of the questions that are asked are specified.

(99) (B) Doctors, researchers, nurses, social workers, or lay people depending on the type of scale.

Some psychiatric rating instruments are designed to be used only by doctoral-level clinicians. Some rating scales can be administered by social workers with clinical experience or psychiatric nurses. Other scales are designed for the layperson without clinical experience or knowledge of psychopathology.

(100) (D) A patient with bipolar disorder currently in a manic episode.

Instruments can obtain information from different sources. The patient who knows the most about his/her condition can be the only source of information. In some situations, the use of an informant is preferable. For example, when the patient has limited insight into their condition (e.g., psychosis or mania), or if the patient has severe social undesirability (e.g., antisocial personality disorder or substance abuse), it is better to use other informants to obtain information.

(101) (C) A 60-year-old patient in a depressive episode.

The clinician does not require an informant when administering a psychiatric rating scale to a patient with a depressive episode. The following situations benefit from the use of an informant: patients with a cognitive disorder, delirium, dementia, or disorders in young children, patients with limited insight (e.g., psychosis, mania), and patients with severe social undesirability (e.g., antisocial personality disorder or substance abuse).

(102) (B) WHO Disability Assessment Schedule cale 2.0 (WHODAS 2.0).

The World Health Association developed the WHO Disability Assessment Schedule scale as the most commonly used scale to measure disability. It is now in its second edition (WHODAS 2.0). This scale is self-administered and it measures several parameters of disability such as interpersonal relations, work impairment, social impairment, cognition, etc. The WHODAS 2.0 can be administered at different intervals throughout the illness. It can track changes that occur as a positive or negative response to a therapeutic intervention.

(103) (A) Positive and Negative Syndrome Scale (PANSS).

The Positive and Negative Syndrome Scale (PANSS) is used to assess positive and negative symptoms of schizophrenia and other psychotic disorders. It is designed for clinicians since it requires clinical judgment. There is a semi-structured interview guide developed for this scale. The PANNS is the gold standard instrument for assessing clinical outcome in studies of schizophrenia treatment. It can be used to track symptom severity in clinical settings.

(104) (A) Bipolar Disorder, current manic episode.

Instruments that are used in the domain of mood disorders assess depression and mania. Patients who are in mania have limited insight and agitation may impair the ability to accurately report symptoms. Therefore, rating scales generally require clinician ratings and data obtained from informants. Depression, however, depends on the patient's subjective experience of their mood state. Interview and self-reporting scales are common in the assessment of depression.

(105) (B) Hamilton Rating Scale for Depression (HAM-D).

The HAM-D is used to measure the symptom severity of major depression and has a focus on somatic complaints. There are versions with different numbers of items, but the most used one is the 17-item version. The HAM-D was originally developed for clinician raters but it can be used by lay administrators. The ratings are completed by the person who is conducting the interview with the patient and their observations.

(106) (C) Patients who suffer from depression and a medical illness.

The HAM-D is used to measure the symptom severity of major depression. It can assess changes in response to health interventions (e.g., pharmacological interventions). It may be problematic to use in elderly patients and patients with medical illnesses since the presence of somatic symptoms in these patients may not be a sign of major depression.

(107) (B) Clinician-Administered PTSD Scale (CAPS).

The CAPS consists of 17 items that cover all four criteria (the event, reexperiencing of the event, avoidance, and increased arousal). It is used to establish the diagnosis of PTSD. The CAPS also includes global rating scales that measure the impact PTSD has on the patient's social and occupational functioning. The CAPS is designed to be administered by a trained clinician. It is used in clinical studies for diagnosis and severity assessment.

(108) (A) Yale-Brown Obsessive-Compulsive Scale (YBOCS).

The YBOCS is a rating scale that measures the severity of OCD symptoms. It consists of ten items. The first five items are related to obsessions such as how much time they consume, to what degree they interfere in the patient's daily functioning, how much distress they cause, how much the patient attempts to resist, and how much the patient is able to control them. The other five items are parallel questions about compulsions.

(109) (A) Beck Depression Inventory (BDI).

The BDI measures depression severity. It mainly focuses on the cognitive and behavioral dimensions of depression. The Beck-II (current version) includes somatic symptoms and the most recent two weeks. Previous versions focus on shorter intervals. The BDI is a self-report instrument that can be completed in five to ten minutes. Its main use is a measurement of outcomes in studies for major depression interventions. The BDI can be used as a screening instrument for major depression.

(110) (D) CAGE.

The CAGE is a short screening instrument for alcohol problems that can be used in various settings. CAGE is an acronym for four questions. A score of one is given to each "yes" answer. A score of one means the person might have an alcohol problem and needs a follow-up. A score of two or more than two suggests significant alcohol problems. The instrument can be completed in less than a minute.

(111) (C) Addiction Severity Index (ASI).

The ASI measures symptoms and functional impairment caused by drug or alcohol abuse. It consists of demographics, drug use, alcohol use, medical status, psychiatric status, employment, family issues, social issues, and legal status. The ASI assesses the duration, frequency, and severity of drug or alcohol use. Both subjective and objective reports by the patient and the interviewer are included.

(112) (C) Time constraints.

The lack of time can be a significant barrier to communication. Rushed meetings are less effective than leisure ones. However, due to the increased demands, nurses may be pressured to neglect the aspect of quality versus quantity. Communication does not always have to be time-consuming. Sometimes, simple "small talk" or a smile may be enough for certain patients.

(113) (D) Explain to the group therapy patients that you must leave and arrange the time when you will be coming back.

In pressured clinics or wards, there may be interruptions or delays in the conversations between healthcare providers and patients. This usually occurs because of the needs of other patients. This may frustrate patients and make them feel neglected. When interruptions happen, it is best to explain to patients why you have to leave and arrange a time for your return.

(114) (C) The background noise.

Sometimes healthcare providers get used to their environment, so they may not notice environmental factors that are causing communication difficulties. Busy clinics with a lot of background noise can impair patients' hearing. Some patients can pretend that they can hear you by nodding. This patient might feel uncomfortable telling you that she is having trouble hearing you. Therefore, you should assume that the background noise is interfering with the effectiveness of communication.

(115) (A) Yelling at the patient.

When you notice that a patient is not hearing well, you should make an effort to reduce the background noise. You can try to find a quiet corner or go to a quieter room. Notice if the patient is wearing any hearing aids, and if they are, check if the hearing aids are working properly. Patients with dementia have cognitive impairments and difficulties with concentration. Noise and distractions can significantly impact communication with these patients.

(116) (C) A 23-year-old Latino patient with Generalized Anxiety Disorder (GAD) who does not understand English very well.

Written forms can be used when patients do not want to disclose sensitive information because they do not want other people to overhear the conversation. Patients will not disclose sensitive information if they feel like other people can hear them. Some patients can have trouble with reading and writing. Some patients who do not understand the language may need someone to translate the form for them.

(117) (B) Acknowledge their discomfort and express that it is important to talk.

Patients who are in distress, or pain, or who are experiencing fatigue may have difficulties with concentration. This can affect the information gathering process. If it is important to obtain information in a moment when a patient is in distress, you can try explaining and acknowledging their discomfort by saying, "I know you are not feeling very well right now, but we must talk."

(118) (A) By breaking down the information into smaller parts.

If patients are unable to give their full attention, try breaking down information into smaller parts so it is easier to digest. Ask patients if they need you to repeat the information. Acknowledging the patient's distress can build rapport and make the patient more communicative. If the information is very important, you can check if the patient understood by asking them to repeat the information back to you.

(119) (D) Blushing.

Patients may feel embarrassed when having to talk about sensitive information like difficult family situations, addictions, sexual dysfunction, etc. Embarrassment can reduce the effectiveness of communication. Blushing is an obvious sign of embarrassment. Other signs include laughter, fidgeting, joking, and other behaviors that aim to mask embarrassment. Use positive and open body language when talking to patients. This will make them feel more comfortable.

(120) (C) When was the last time you had a glass of wine?

You should avoid judgmental statements since they increase embarrassment. This can be seen in the way you phrase questions as well. Asking the patient when they last had a glass of wine is a more neutral and open way to ask for information and it will elicit a more honest answer.

(121) (C) Patients have no issues asking for clarifications when they have trouble understanding something.

Patients may feel reluctant to ask for clarification since they may feel like they are wasting their time. You should let them know that taking care of their health is your job and that there are no stupid questions. You can encourage them to ask questions by saying, "I know you have questions. Is there anything that you would like me to answer for you?"

(122) (B) To make communication between healthcare providers easier.

Technical jargon and clinical acronyms are helpful in the communication between healthcare providers. However, you should remember to avoid using technical jargon in front of patients. This requires conscious effort since it is easy to slip jargon into a conversation without noticing it. When patients hear technical terms, they may be reluctant to admit that they do not understand what has been said.

(123) (C) Talking slowly.

If the patient is not fluent in English, avoid complex sentences and slang, and try to speak more slowly. Avoid talking about statistics since this may be confusing for most patients. You should try to avoid using ambiguous terms since some words have one meaning for you but may have a different meaning for the patient. The vocabulary should be appropriate for the specific audience. Do not use childish expressions with elderly patients.

(124) (A) Introduce himself and his role.

Everyone has different assumptions, values, cultural beliefs, biases, and prejudices. Some patients may find it hard to believe that a man can be a nurse or that a doctor can be a female. Notice assumptions that can cause misinterpretations. Sometimes assumptions may cause a patient to ignore you. You can solve these situations by introducing yourself and your role by saying, "Hello, I am your mental health nurse practitioner and I will be examining you today."

(125) (D) Calling the patient at random times during the day if you remember additional information.

When you need to provide the patient with a lot of new information, you can ask the patient to bring a family member or a friend, so they can both hear it. You can tell the patient they can take notes if they wish. You can record the conversation so they can hear it again at a later time. Calling the patient might make them uncomfortable and disturb their day.

(126) (C) Speed of speech, intonation, voice quality, and rhythm.

Cultural norms and customs influence the way we think and the way we express ourselves. Expression of communication is done through language (speaking and writing), paralanguage (speed of speech, intonation, voice quality, rhythm), and gestures (facial expression, body posture, eye movements, physical appearance, touch). When there is a language barrier between a healthcare provider and the patient, an interpreter might be necessary.

(127) (B) Speaking to the interpreter and not directly to the patient.

When using an interpreter, you should speak directly to the patient instead of speaking to the interpreter. Maintain eye contact with the patient to keep them involved. When the patient and interpreter are talking, do not interrupt them. Their interactions may require more time since there may be dialect differences or a need for more extensive clarifications.

(128) (A) You should use technical jargon when talking to the interpreter.

Avoid using technical jargon which may be difficult for both patient and interpreter to understand. Avoid long conversations with the interpreter in front of the patient since this can make the patient feel left out and ignored. You should instruct the interpreter to translate in the same words as the patient so you can understand what the patient is thinking and feeling.

(129) (A) To be of the same gender and similar age as the patient.

Use an interpreter who is the same age and similar age as the patient. If there is a possibility, you can allow the patient and interpreter to meet before the interview to build rapport. This can be positive for the interview. If it's possible, use the same interpreter for subsequent interviews with the same patient.

(130) (C) Failures occur because of external circumstances.

In collectivist cultures, individuals often attribute their failures to external circumstances rather than personal deficiencies. This perspective emphasizes the influence of the environment and external factors on an individual's outcomes.

(131) (C) Patients with different cultural backgrounds use the same terms to describe mental illness.

Different cultural groups have different languages and may have different terms for mental health issues. Factors that motivate communication, such as rules and rituals, also vary between different cultural groups.

(132) (B) Behavioral symptoms in dementia.

The NPI is used to assess behavioral symptoms seen in Alzheimer's disease and other types of dementia. It assesses twelve areas: apathy, aberrant motor behavior, appetite, anxiety, agitation/aggression, delusions, dysphoria, disinhibition, delusions, euphoria, irritability/lability, nocturnal disturbances, and eating. It can be completed in fifteen to twenty minutes. The NPI is used in both research and clinical settings.

(133) (D) The Mini-Mental State Examination (MMSE) is a cognitive test that is used to assess cognitive functions in many domains (orientation, memory, language, attention, and construction).

The MMSE is a cognitive test that consists of 30 points. It is used to assess cognitive functions in many domains (orientation, memory, language, attention, and construction). Any decline in general intelligence can be a sign of a cognitive disorder and requires further work-up.

(134) (D) Imperfections of processes and systems.

Factors involved in the complexity of healthcare include inefficient processes, variability in health insurance, differences in education and experience of providers, variability in patient populations, and many others. A quality healthcare system should be safe, efficient, effective, timely, equitable, and patient-centered. Healthcare quality should be measured to assess the impact of healthcare on the desired outcomes and determine whether healthcare professionals adhere to processes that are based on scientific evidence and consistent with patient preferences.

(135) (A) The number of nurses with appropriate education and training, the number of beds in the hospital, and health insurance.

The structure includes the number of nurses with appropriate education and training, the number of beds in the hospital, and health insurance. When measuring the process, assessment is done on the delivery of healthcare services by healthcare providers, such as the usage of up-to-date guidelines for the care of patients with anxiety disorders. The measurement of outcomes refers to the result of healthcare which is impacted by both behavioral and environmental factors.

(136) (B) Continuous Quality Improvement.

Continuous quality improvement (CQI) is used interchangeably with Total Quality Improvement (TQM). The CQI approach is based on the premise that to achieve the best outcome, the whole organization should commit to quality. It states that every process can be improved. The CQI approach is used to develop clinical practice. In-hospital quality assurance (QA) programs are focused on problems identified by accreditation or regulatory organizations.

(137) (C) Incorporation of beliefs and values in the improvement process.

Clinical practice improvement (CPI) is an approach that aims to implement change in the healthcare delivery process to achieve the best outcomes in the clinical management of patients. Quality improvement processes focus on identifying a process that needs to be improved, measuring the factors involved in key performance, conducting a detailed analysis to develop a new approach, integrating the new approach with the process, and reassessments to determine whether the change has resulted in an improved process.

(138) (C) Incorporating reminders in charts for providers.

Examples of quality improvement strategies and tools include providing reminder systems by incorporating reminders in charts for providers, developing computer-based reminders, and computer-based decision support; providing audit and feedback by giving performance feedback to individual providers, incorporating quality indicators and reports, publicly releasing performance data, and incorporating National/State quality report cards; education of providers by including them in workshops and conferences, distributing educational material and content, and initiating educational outreach visits.

(139) (B) The Plan-Do-Study-Act (PDSA)

The Plan-Do-Study-Act (PDSA) model aims to improve quality, make positive changes in healthcare, and achieve favorable outcomes. This model has a rapid cyclical nature and accomplishes change through regular and small PDSAs. The main purpose of PDSA is to demonstrate a relationship between process changes (e.g., behaviors and capabilities) and outcomes.

(140) (C) Adverse events are overreported.

Adverse events can be prevented by identifying the points in the healthcare process that are prone to mistakes and changing these processes in a way that will reduce the likelihood of harm. This requires obtaining data on preventable adverse events, which remain grossly underreported. The Institute of Medicine (IOM) recommends systematic reporting of healthcare errors and adverse events to improve patient safety.

(141) (C) Healthcare providers do not have public accountability to provide information about their performance and actions to the public.

Healthcare providers have public accountability to provide information about their performance and actions to the public. Oversight bodies exist to make sure that providers are compliant with accepted standards of care. When an adverse event occurs, oversight bodies should investigate the causes behind it. This information improves public safety.

(142) (B) It should be significantly influenced by the clinician's education.

An event should be clearly measurable and identifiable. The event's occurrence should be significantly influenced by the healthcare facility's procedures and policies. The event should pose a concern to the public and healthcare providers. The event should be serious, unambiguous, and preventable. It should indicate a problem in the safety systems of the healthcare facility, and it should have importance for public accountability or credibility.

(143) (B) Healthcare facilities should eliminate all risk of adverse events.

Healthcare facilities are not able to eliminate the risk of adverse events. However, they can take actions and measures that will reduce that risk. The list consists of twenty-seven serious reportable adverse events. They are organized into six categories. Five categories are related to the provision of care (e.g., care management, environmental, patient protection, product or device, and surgical), while one includes criminal events.

(144) (C) The clinician's ethnic background.

Patients have expectations of what will be required of them, what the likely outcome is, how much time it will take to achieve that outcome, the clinician's responsibilities, the relationship between the clinician and the patient, and others. Factors that influence patient expectations include the patient's personality, previous experiences with mental health treatment, whether treatment is voluntary or involuntary, and what kind of information they have obtained through the media or others.

(145) (C) Therapeutic behavioral techniques.

Patients who have suffered a stroke may be limited in mobility due to paralysis. This may impair their ability to use behavioral techniques. If the stroke has resulted in speech deficits, these patients may have difficulties with therapeutic techniques that involve verbal expression.

(146) (A) Cognitive Behavioral Therapy.

Cognitive Behavioral Therapy involves verbal expression where patients discuss their thoughts and feelings. It focuses on identifying and changing negative thought patterns and behaviors through structured conversations and activities.

(147) (D) Healthcare providers have become more sensitive to psychiatric issues in their patients.

Healthcare providers (physicians, clinical nurse practitioners, physician assistants) in nonpsychiatric medical professions have become more sensitive to psychiatric issues in their patients. Because of this, the number of referrals to psychiatry has increased. This means that healthcare providers in psychiatry are seeing more patients with comorbid medical conditions. Therefore, healthcare providers should be educated in common physical diseases and disorders and consider them in the treatment plan development.

(148) (B) Clinical practice guidelines.

Clinical practice guidelines are systematically developed declarations that support certain treatment actions or approaches. Guidelines are a representation of a consensus of experts who have agreed upon what the best treatment approach is for a certain patient under specific circumstances.

(149) (C) They tend to involve mechanical implementation which makes them inflexible and nonintuitive.

A treatment manual may not meet the patient's needs and may limit the healthcare provider's actions. Treatment manuals have a negative impact on the doctor-patient relationship. However, they can be used to train therapists in specific models, reduce variability between practices, and facilitate greater patient involvement in treatment.

(150) (D) Empirically Supported Treatments.

Empirically supported treatments integrate the best available research combined with clinical experience. Empirically supported treatments have demonstrated effectiveness and achievement of positive outcomes in randomized controlled trials. There are many empirically supported treatments developed for mental health issues, such as cognitive behavioral therapy (CBT) or interpersonal psychotherapy.

Download the Exam Simulator Instructions, Additional Tests, and Other Files!

Scan the QR code below with your phone and you will be given a link to Google Drive where you can download the files.

If the QR code does not work for you, please contact us at info@newstonetestprep.com and mention the title of this book.